The HIV-Negative Gay Man: Developing Strategies for Survival and Emotional Well-Being

The HIV-Negative Gay Man: Developing Strategies for Survival and Emotional Well-Being has been co-published simultaneously as *Journal of Gay & Lesbian Social Services*, Volume 8, Number 1 1998.

The HIV-Negative Gay Man: Developing Strategies for Survival and Emotional Well-Being

Steven Ball, MA, MSW, ACSW
Editor

The HIV-Negative Gay Man: Developing Strategies for Survival and Emotional Well-Being, edited by Steven Ball, was simultaneously issued by The Haworth Press, Inc., under the same title, as a special issue of Journal of Gay & Lesbian Social Services, Volume 8, Number 1 1998, James J. Kelly, Editor.

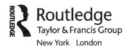

Routledge
Taylor & Francis Group
New York   London

1-56023-114-9

First Published by

The Harrington Park Press, 10 Alice Street, Binghamton, NY 13904-1580 USA

The Harrington Park Press is an imprint of The Haworth Press, Inc., 10 Alice Street, Binghamton, NY 13904-1580 USA.

This edition published 2012 by Routledge

Routledge
Taylor & Francis Group
711 Third Avenue
New York, NY 10017

Routledge
Taylor & Francis Group
2 Park Square, Milton Park
Abingdon, Oxon, OX14 4RN

The HIV-Negative Gay Man: Developing Strategies for Survival and Emotional Well-Being **has been co-published simultaneously as *Journal of Gay & Lesbian Social Services,* Volume 8, Number 1 1998.**

The development, preparation, and publication of this work has been undertaken with great care. However, the publisher, employees, editors, and agents of The Haworth Press and all imprints of The Haworth Press, Inc., including The Haworth Medical Press and The Pharmaceutical Products Press, are not responsible for any errors contained herein or for consequences that may ensue from use of materials or information contained in this work. Opinions expressed by the author(s) are not necessarily those of The Haworth Press, Inc.

Cover design by Marylouise E. Doyle

Library of Congress Cataloging-in-Publication Data

HIV-negative gay man : developing strategies for survival and emotional well-being / Steven Ball, editor.
     p. cm.
     "The HIV-negative gay man : developing strategies for survival and emotional well-being has been co-published simultaneously as Journal of gay & lesbian social services, volume 8, number 1, 1998"–T.p. verso.
     Includes bibliographical references and index.
     ISBN 0-7890-0522-0 (alk. paper). - ISBN 1-56023-114-9 (pbk.: alk. paper)
     1. AIDS (Disease)–Social aspects. 2. AIDS (Disease)–Psychological aspects. 3. Gay men–Diseases. 4. Gay men–Mental health. I. Ball, Steven. II. Title: Journal of gay and lesbian social services, v. 8, no. 1.
RA644.A25H588 1998
362.1 '969792–dc21
                                        98-12623
                                           CIP

For Michael whose faith in me and ongoing passionate support helped nurture this book

And to Ben . . . for everything

CONTENTS

ABOUT THE EDITOR

Steven Ball, MA, MSW, ACSW is a social worker and psychotherapist in private practice in New York City. For the past decade he has specialized in developing group interventions for marginalized members of the gay community. He is currently a consultant to the HIV Prevention Department at Gay Men's Health Crisis, the oldest and largest AIDS service organization in the world, where he is supervising the development of time limited groups for gay men who are HIV negative, and is a frequent speaker at national conferences, and the author of numerous articles on working with gay men. He is also a drama therapist with an expertise in working with geriatric and persistently mentally ill populations.

Foreword

Today any mental health professional who works with large numbers of gay men hears and must address the variety and complexity of emotional reactions of gay men who are HIV negative to living in a community under assault by AIDS. When Walt Odets (1995) began to alert both the general and mental health communities to the realities that men uninfected with HIV have unique psychosocial issues that must be worked through if their emotional health and well being is to be sustained, his ideas and work were reviled and dismissed by many within the gay men's community. There were public declarations that HIV negative men were "whiners" or merely "worried well." Since they were uninfected they did not really have anything to complain about. Some people living with HIV and AIDS were outraged by the assertion that uninfected men had important struggles that also needed to be addressed in order to insure a good quality of life not just for men like them who are infected, but for all of the gay community.

Michael Shernoff, MSW, is a therapist in private practice in Manhattan, and adjunct lecturer at Hunter College Graduate School of Social Work. He has edited *The Sourcebook on Lesbian/Gay Health Care, Volumes 1 and 2, Counseling Chemically Dependent People With HIV Illness* and *Human Services for Gay People: Clinical and Community Practice* and coedited (with Walt Odets) *The Second Decade of AIDS: A Mental Health Practice Handbook.* He is a contributing editor to *In the Family* magazine, and a senior consulting editor at the *Journal of Gay & Lesbian Social Services.* His most recent book, *Gay Widowers: Life After the Death of a Partner,* was published in December 1997 by The Harrington Park Press (E-mail: mshernoff @aol.com or at his home page http://members.aol.com/therapysvc/index.html).

[Haworth co-indexing entry note]: "Foreword." Shernoff, Michael. Co-published simultaneously in *Journal of Gay & Lesbian Social Services* (The Haworth Press, Inc.) Vol. 8, No. 1, 1998, pp. xvii-xxvii; and: *The HIV-Negative Gay Man: Developing Strategies for Survival and Emotional Well-Being* (ed: Steven Ball) The Haworth Press, Inc., 1998, pp. xiii-xxiii; and: *The HIV-Negative Gay Man: Developing Strategies for Survival and Emotional Well-Being* (ed: Steven Ball) The Harrington Park Press, an imprint of The Haworth Press, Inc., 1998, pp. xiii-xxiii. Single or multiple copies of this article are available for a fee from The Haworth Document Delivery Service [1-800-342-9678, 9:00 a.m. - 5:00 p.m. (EST). E-mail address: getinfo@haworth.com].

As both a psychotherapist and an HIV positive individual, I have recognized for many years the validity of what Odets described, and am saddened by assertions that providing services to the uninfected dilutes efforts to help people who are living with HIV or AIDS. I am concerned that few if any HIV positive professionals or individuals have rallied to identify and provide services for men who are not infected. Uninfected men have been providing services both in volunteer and professional capacities for people with HIV/AIDS since the onset of the epidemic, and it behooves all of us, infected and uninfected alike, to do everything in our power to ensure that no one else becomes infected.

The current divisions in the gay men's community between men who are negative and those who are infected with HIV or ill with AIDS is not new. This division takes many forms. Some positive men, for example, only want to date other positive men and some negative men refuse to go out with anyone who has not tested HIV negative. Historically there have been many efforts on the part of some gay men to distance themselves from other gay men who were different from them. In the very early days of attempting to get a gay rights bill passed by the New York City council, for instance, opponents of the bill asserted that if the bill were to pass, drag queens would be permitted to teach in the schools. (Heaven forbid!!) Some gay activists felt that as a strategy to try and get the bill passed, it would be acceptable to delete protection for transvestites. This position caused a major uproar and was soon abandoned. People who are not into the leather or s/m scenes are embarrassed by the public displays of the leather sexuality at gay pride marches and voice their concerns that only "normal looking" gay people should be public. On certain levels, the split between infected and uninfected men is often nothing more than a continuation of a pattern of distancing oneself from people whom it is threatening to view as, in fact, quite similar to oneself. Responding to concerns of all members is essential for the survival of a vibrant gay men's community.

Both the successes and failures of the early AIDS prevention efforts must necessarily influence the new efforts for keeping men uninfected. Thirteen years ago when I coauthored the first generation of safer sex interventions for gay and bisexual men beginning with the "Hot, Horny & Healthy: Eroticizing Safer Sex" workshops, I never dreamed that more than a decade later the AIDS plague would still be decimating the gay men's community. In the mid 1980s most of us doing prevention work with gay men did not have an inkling that there would still be a dire need for prevention programs to help gay men remain uninfected many years after our initial AIDS prevention efforts. But the tragic reality is that HIV and AIDS have become a permanent part of our emotional, social, and sexual landscapes, requiring that a series of essays like this be written.

In the early days of the AIDS epidemic, I failed to grasp that the behavior changes I was attempting to help gay men adopt would need to become permanent and life long. Ah, if I were only able to recapture some of the naivete of those days! Those initial workshops were designed as an immediate response to a sexually transmitted health crisis. I firmly believed then, and continue to believe now, that only by celebrating the normalcy and healthiness of gay men's needs for social, emotional, and sexual connections with each other could we begin to help men not place themselves or others at risk of becoming infected. When gay men deeply feel good about themselves, good about what they do sexually, and good about their partners, there is a hope and possibility that they will choose not to behave in ways that will continue to transmit HIV. All AIDS prevention efforts aimed at gay men must be unapologetically sex positive and gay positive. This is critically important to help ameliorate the negative impact that a sexually transmitted epidemic is having on many gay men by reinforcing preexisting internalized homophobia and erotophobia. In addition, the centrality of sex as one of the ordinary and essential expressions of our love for each other must never be minimized or under valued.

We have come a long way since the first excruciatingly frightening days of learning how to live with AIDS as an unwelcome intruder in our lives and community. We now know much more about how HIV is transmitted, and there is probably not a gay man alive who doesn't know that anal sex without a condom is a high risk activity. Yet thousands of men still choose to engage in this behavior, even with men they know are HIV positive or whose HIV status they do not know. It is important not to simply pathologize men who knowingly engage in high risk sexual behaviors, nor seek out simplistic explanations that unsafe sexual behaviors are only an expression of low self-esteem or occur solely under the influence of alcohol or drugs. Nobody expected to have to change the way they had gay sex for the rest of their lives, and therein lies part of the explanation for new infections.

Immediately after the fact that HIV was sexually transmitted became general knowledge, some men simply attempted to refrain from sex in an effort to protect themselves from infection. Invariably the men who chose to stop having sex in response to AIDS began to report that periodically they would finally give in to their urge for sex, and indulge in a variety of sexual acts, some of which were unsafe. Wracked by both guilt and fear at having done high risk behaviors, these men vowed "never to do it again!" Obviously this was a highly unrealistic declaration. Among therapists and AIDS prevention specialists this kind of behavior soon became known as a "diet/binge sexual syndrome," and made clear that gay men needed to integrate ways of making the necessary behavior changes within the context of remaining sexually active. Thus the early interventions addressed men discovering that the possibility for remaining sexually active and sexually satisfied within the limitations of safer sex did in fact exist. As we have sadly learned in the ensuing years, by not addressing the emotional and social realities of sex in the lives of gay men, we were limiting the long term effectiveness of those important early interventions.

In his book *Reviving the Tribe*, long time community activist Eric Rofes (1996) chides the structures of our multifaceted community and culture that with "few exceptions, seem hell bent on avoiding the depth of the impact of the epidemic" (p. 25). He describes the reverberations that the decimation of two generations of gay men is having on a community level. He poses questions about why outside of therapy offices there remained an absence of forums in which open discussion within the community about these realities took place. He states that "until recently, I believed that the epidemic's impact on gay male culture had been limited to our intimate, interpersonal and communal relations–as well as hundreds of thousands of lives. But I have come to believe that we have our own 'corpses of history' as poignant and meaningful to us as specific burned out shells of landmarks were to residents of cities that experienced mass bombings during WWII" (Rofes, 1996, p. 32). Both Rofes and Odets link this community denial and frustration to partly explain why some gay men knowingly put themselves at risk for becoming infected with HIV. It is exactly this mega-impact of AIDS on HIV negative gay men and the development of environmental, communal and therapeutic interventions to provide forums for negative men to begin to have their needs met that is described in the following essays. This collection presents the cutting edge, state of the art efforts at preventing new cases of HIV infection among gay men today.

As someone who designed several of the initial safe sex interventions for gay and bisexual men, and has been a long term nonprogressor living with HIV for many years, I now have a crucial understanding of why brief, psychoeducational behavioral workshops are no longer able to help gay men stay uninfected in the second decade of the epidemic. In my practice I work daily with men who struggle to overcome a life long legacy of homonegativity. Combined with the devastating psychic impact that more than a decade of living under the shadow of AIDS has introduced, it is truly remarkable that any gay man has not succumbed to despair but rather strives to challenge himself to create meaningful relationships and a satisfying life.

Many of the psychodynamic and interpersonal issues of asymptomatic but infected gay men mirror those of HIV negative gay men. I often ponder "why have I been spared when so many others became sick, deteriorated and died?" Personally I do not suffer from the survivor guilt that is similar to what many HIV negative men are experiencing, but I know asymptomatic HIV infected men who are unable to unambivalently rejoice in their good fortune. HIV negative gay men are often wracked by fears that perhaps they will not remain uninfected. I am often consumed with fears that perhaps my continued good health will suddenly change for the worse. Like HIV negative gay men I feel alone with these feelings and concerns and have few places and people with whom to discuss them outside of my therapy. It would certainly seem indulgent to share these feelings with friends who are symptomatic and struggling with the ravages of full blown AIDS. Yet there is an urgency and poignancy in what I live with on a daily basis that is remarkably similar to what I hear HIV negative friends and patients discuss. All these similarities between uninfected and long term nonprogressors reaffirm why the community-wide attention to the issues discussed in this book are crucial for the continued survival and well being of a robust gay men's community. As a community that was initially under siege by homophobia, hatred and discrimination, and now additionally by a rampant virus, we do not have the luxury of ignoring the differences as well as similarities that exist between men of different sero-statuses.

Some men may simply place priority on quality of pleasure over longevity of life. "The role of both AIDS education and prevention is to make certain that gay men have all of the information about the risks of various sexual behaviors so they can make individually informed and responsible choices. In addition programs need to simultaneously attempt to help all generations of gay men discover the potential for having a meaningful life despite the harsh and unrelenting realities of AIDS so they will more often choose to make decisions that ensure their survival" (Rofes, 1996, p. 210). Thus what is needed are holistic environmental approaches to AIDS education and prevention which go way beyond primary emphasis on safer sex. These macro, community-wide interventions must help gay men struggle with the options for attaining a desired high quality of life in the midst of this ongoing threat. In order to do this the programs have to be unapologetic in promoting sex and love between men that can only begin when men value communication, honesty, and mutuality in their relationships with one another. These are the qualities inherent in the programs many of the authors of the various essays in this collection describe.

What has been lacking in so many of the AIDS prevention efforts that have come before the ones described in this collection, has been a thorough exploration of the meaning of various gay male sexual activities such as: the importance for some men to have a man inside of them without a condom; some gay men experience receiving (or giving) of semen as an intimate and possibly sacred act; and many men have a powerful desire for penetration and receiving semen. Existing priorities which place prevention, halting transmission, and survival by any means necessary, must be superseded by education, empowerment, and acceptance of the diverse ways men will come to terms with life in the epidemic.

The ongoing nature of the AIDS epidemic has colored all aspects of life for contemporary gay men that is virtually incomprehensible to those who are not affected. This reality brings new challenges, dynamics, and skills to psychotherapy, counseling, mental health, and social services for gay men. As several of the essays in this collection so aptly illustrate, no gay man doing clinical work with other gay men in this the age of AIDS, can indulge in the illusion of objectivity or distance from clients who are discussing the multiple ways that AIDS affects their lives and psyches.

If the practitioner is himself infected that brings its own set of issues, and complications that must be dealt with, ideally in any form of supervision, in order to both ensure that the treatment remains correctly focused as well as to protect both the clinician and the client from understandable potential complications. If the provider is negative, then he is living with the same feelings and uncertainties as his negative clients. AIDS and its unforeseen changes and influences are necessitating the formulation of a homo-centric perspective to working with today's gay men. This perspective must incorporate an understanding of the totality that the impact of AIDS is having on all gay men. No area of gay men's existence is untouched by the reality that AIDS has been decimating our community for more than a decade, and, with the new infection rates, this catastrophe shows no indication of abating. Dynamics of loss, sadness, helplessness, hopelessness, powerlessness, despair, grief, and trauma, combined with heroism, selflessness, and human sacrifice are constantly at play in the psyches and daily lives of all gay men.

It is often overwhelming to have a confirmed exposure to HIV for more than twenty years, have remained in perfect health and to have witnessed the deaths of almost my entire circle of friends, my beloved partner, numerous acquaintances, and more than 150 patients. Immersing myself in providing mental health services to people with HIV/AIDS, designing prevention programs, and training other professionals around the United States, was partly an attempt to mitigate my own sense of helplessness and powerlessness about changing the outcome of this horrible illness. During the course of the AIDS epidemic I have left my youth behind and entered middle age. As I look around, too many of the men who would have been sharing middle age with me are now gone. Thus I was thrilled when several years ago Steve Ball began to talk and consult with me regarding the HIV negative groups he had developed initially for The Manhattan Center for Living. Finally someone was doing something to help those lucky enough to have thus far escaped infection. What the groups described in this book really consist of are community mental health interventions that now need to become institutionalized on a broad basis.

I dream of the day when this disease is truly a chronic and manageable illness. I do not believe that in my life time we will see either a vaccine or a cure, although I fervently hope that I am short sighted and incorrect in these beliefs! The pragmatist in me does not allow me to dare to envision a day when nobody else will become infected. But validating and empowering HIV negative gay men will certainly go far to making certain that we can reduce the numbers of men who do become infected.

The efforts described in the essays compiled by Steven Ball pose thrilling challenges for all of us who love the gay community in general and gay men specifically. "A change in prevention strategy may lead us to assume a broader mission, focused on assisting a gay population besieged by death and discrimination to create forms of life that are worth living. An emphasis on quality of life, rather than length of life, may offer a modicum of hope and engagement now lacking; simultaneously it also may support a prevention agenda and ultimately lead to reduced HIV transmission. Reconceptualizing work with gay men's sex opens many new questions. Rather than inquiring, 'How can we educate gay men to have only safe sex?' or 'Can we shift peer pressure so as to influence private as well as public acts?' we need to ask 'How can gay men create lives worth living?' or 'What can the community offer to gay men which is engaging, affirming, and life-sustaining?' " (Rofes, 1996, pp. 210-211). The articles that follow describe attempts to provide uninfected gay men with venues where they can begin to develop strategies that contribute to the regeneration of the potential for gay men to have a sense of well being in the midst of the epidemic and optimism about the ability of gay male culture and community to continue to develop as we approach the twenty-first century. It requires the acknowledgment that gay men as a class do not embrace a single answer to the existential questions posed by the catastrophe of AIDS.

Steven Ball is a pioneer in helping HIV negative gay men survive this plague. He needs to be acknowledged for being the person who first organized groups for HIV negative gay men in New York City beginning in January 1994 first through The Manhattan Center for Living, then in his private practice and eventually at Gay Men's Health Crisis. He is also to be commended for his leadership and vision in bringing together the current collection of essays.

The first community-wide effort to address the impact of AIDS on uninfected gay men that I know about occurred in Boston in 1991 when the Fenway Community Health Center organized a community forum on the issue that was attended by more than ninety men. Out of this meeting the first ongoing facilitated groups for HIV negative gay men were organized (Johnston, 1995). Three years later, at about the same time that the groups for HIV negative gay men were first being organized in New York by Steve Ball, two clinicians in Los Angeles were forming ongoing groups for this population. Steve Buckingham of The AIDS Project Los Angeles and Ian Stulberg of The AIDS Services Center of Pasadena began a twelve week group model in a joint project between those two agencies. The AIDS Services Center continues to run these groups and they are well attended. Initially in New York, Boston, and San Francisco, groups for HIV negative gay men were far from fashionable, and were often criticized for taking the focus off "the people with real serious issues of living with HIV and AIDS." Interestingly, in Los Angeles and New York the provision of services for uninfected men did not cause the outcry from people living with HIV and AIDS that it did in San Francisco.

The authors of the essays in this collection provide anyone concerned with helping gay men remain uninfected with HIV with provocative and thoughtful material. These authors comprise the contemporary vanguard of gay affirmative psychotherapists. They continue the historic tradition of those first pioneers who in the 1970s were lonely voices articulating and advocating that there was a need for specific mental health and social services for gay people that was not aimed at changing an individual's sexual orientation.

Today we take it for granted that sexual minority communities should have the opportunity and in fact need, to have access to sympathetic and well trained professionals who value their being different from mainstream society. But this development has come about in less than twenty years. Even today, in certain professional circles gay affirmative services are still looked on with distrust and are viewed as an aberration. I am pleased that providing services to HIV negative gay men is no longer controversial and is becoming fully integrated into the field of gay affirmative psychotherapy and counseling, as one respected and essential component of the full range of social services.

In the early days of gay affirmative mental health services, both professionals and peer counselors spent hours in supervision addressing the impact that our being similar to our clients had on the provision of good quality services. There was an urgency and immediacy to the issues brought to us by our clients that mirrored our own personal and professional struggles. We learned that, and eventually grew comfortable with the knowledge that it was precisely these similarities that enabled us to have greater empathy for our clients as well as insight into the problems we were being consulted about. The essays that follow illustrate what early feminist theorists taught, "that the personal is still political," or in this case that "the personal is still very much therapeutic." The very lack of separation between the authors of the following essays and the men they work with mirrors many of the struggles experienced by the first wave of clients, peer counselors, and professionals who created gay affirmative psychotherapy. Peer counseling was and remains one important aspect to gay affirmative mental health services all around the United States. The groups run at Gay Men's Health Crisis that are described in several of the following essays (Frederick & Glassman, Ball, Klotz, & Locke) illustrate how peer counselors remain an important and useful resource, continuing a valuable historic tradition within the gay community. Almost all of the authors describe an urgency and immediacy about their work that arises out of the similarities between the issues that clients raise and their own personal realities. The contemporary similarities between HIV negative service providers and clients, and the resulting confusion and discomfort for openly gay providers has long and proud roots in the historic tradition of gay affirmative counseling.

All the authors are to be applauded for "going where no one has gone before." They are brave, skilled, visionary men and clinicians who have my respect and admiration. The essays in this collection are a critically important compilation of efforts to concretely address the variety of psychosocial and psychosexual needs of uninfected gay men. It is only by increasing the kinds of programs described in the following pages that we will ensure the survival of increasing numbers of what the late author Paul Monette often lovingly referred to as "our tribe."

Michael Shernoff

REFERENCES

Johnston, W. (1995). *HIV negative: How the uninfected are affected by AIDS.* New York: Plenum Press.

Odets, W. (1995). *In the shadow of the epidemic: Being HIV negative in the age of AIDS.* Durham, North Carolina: Duke University Press.

Rofes, E. (1996). *Reviving the tribe: Regenerating gay men's sexuality and culture in the ongoing epidemic.* The Harrington Park Press.

PERSONAL PERSPECTIVES

Coming Out in the AIDS Era:
One HIV-Negative Gay Man's Story

Carl Locke

SUMMARY. HIV continues to hold a unique place within the gay male community in the United States. HIV/AIDS has become merged with personal, social, and sexual identities in gay men in ways not replicated in other social groups. Young gay men who have come out since the mid-80s up to today, must do so in an environment where HIV and gay identity are merged. Sexual exploration and a growing sense of belonging to a community coincide with the struggle to remain uninfected with HIV. This is no easy task when we begin to examine the urban gay community, seroprevalance rates, and the unconscious connections to HIV and gay men. This article is a personal story describing a young gay man's struggle with coming out during the era of AIDS and confronting these difficult issues. *[Article copies available for a fee from The Haworth Document Delivery Service: 1-800-342-9678. E-mail address: getinfo@haworth.com]*

Carl Locke, MSW, is Coordinator of Counseling Services at the Geffen Center at Gay Men's Health Crisis. He can be reached at 119 West 24 Street, New York, NY 10011 (E-mail: CarlLocke@aol.com (or) 2Carl@GMHC.org).

[Haworth co-indexing entry note]: "Coming Out in the AIDS Era: One HIV-Negative Gay Man's Story." Locke, Carl. Co-published simultaneously in *Journal of Gay & Lesbian Social Services* (The Haworth Press, Inc.) Vol. 8, No. 1, 1998, pp. 1-12; and: *The HIV-Negative Gay Man: Developing Strategies for Survival and Emotional Well-Being* (ed: Steven Ball) The Haworth Press, Inc., 1998, pp. 1-12; and: *The HIV-Negative Gay Man: Developing Strategies for Survival and Emotional Well-Being* (ed: Steven Ball) The Harrington Park Press, an imprint of The Haworth Press, Inc., 1998, pp. 1-12. Single or multiple copies of this article are available for a fee from The Haworth Document Delivery Service [1-800-342-9678, 9:00 a.m. - 5:00 p.m. (EST). E-mail address: getinfo@haworth.com].

It's 1990. The AIDS epidemic has been raging for nine years. I became involved three years earlier while in my freshman year at Sarah Lawrence College by forming its AIDS Peer Education Project (APE). I left Sarah Lawrence when I should have been beginning my junior year to take a job as a "personal assistant" for a man in New York City who had AIDS. I was his buddy, medication monitor and dispenser, private duty nursing aide for numerous hospitalizations, and just about anything else he needed. My background as a nursing assistant and AIDS educator, plus the connection through a friend, got me the job. Having done AIDS prevention work for the previous two years, I was convinced this kind of direct, hands-on experience with AIDS was what I needed to do next. It didn't hurt that I was going to go to Beverly Hills for the winter to care for Larry in his home there. We never got to Beverly Hills because he became too ill. I managed to find an apartment in New York and worked six days a week for him until he died in November 1989, three months after I began my one year contract with him. Being a boy from rural Virginia, attending college was what I thought I should do to pull myself out of a dismal future. I surprised even myself when I left Sarah Lawrence for this experience.

So, I managed to enroll for the spring semester and was back in college. I continued coordinating the APE, but switched my studies from performing arts to developmental and social psychology. In a zealous attempt to graduate on-time, I took extra courses, one of which was an independent study on Death and Dying. In one of my assignments, I faced a personal dilemma that stunned me and has since shifted my thoughts about myself as a gay man. The paper was on the social impact of multiple deaths from AIDS on the gay community at large. My dilemma surfaced when I tried to write about my role in the gay community. I was surprised because it was the first time I wondered why I was so involved in the epidemic when I did not know anyone personally who had HIV or AIDS, did not personally know anyone who had died from AIDS (I did not consider Larry a personal connection), and did not have HIV myself. In a matter of two years, I had given up my life dream of being a performer for something I wasn't sure how it could become my career. Where was my personal connection and what was driving me? More directly, where was I supposed to go from here? Back at school with three semesters left, what was I going to "be when I grew up?" And how was I part of "the community" and "the fight" if I didn't have HIV?

While writing this article, I realized my questions were not ones that I alone was grappling with, but had ramifications for many young gay men who had come out and became sexual in the midst of the AIDS epidemic. I was struck by the realization that coming-out as a gay man for me was actualized publicly by becoming involved in AIDS work. At the time, the only way I made sense out of this was to look for my own losses on a different level than that of older gay men. I thought about how walking through Greenwich Village would be different if thousands of gay men had not died in the last nine years; about all of the people I could have met but wouldn't; the friends and lovers I would never have; the impact on my relationships with other men who were obviously changed from living through the epidemic; and all of the lost opportunities. I invented my own losses in order to claim a place in the gay community. This was the way I found a fit for myself.

It wasn't until recently that I realized the impact this process would have on me and how profound it would be. Becoming involved in AIDS was my way to declare myself a proud gay man. The AIDS crisis was my vehicle to come out as gay. As much as the gay community did to make the public realize AIDS was not a gay disease, it was the acceptable and action-oriented way I "became gay." It was around AIDS activism that vast numbers of urban gay men met, socialized, made friends, found support, and lived out being gay. Many rural gay boys come to urban meccas to come out and find others like themselves. This is an essential step in the formation of gay identity. While coming out, I found this community, like many others before me, and it helped me greatly in accepting myself and my sexuality. However, a striking difference from any previous time is that the community was merged with AIDS. Because of this, on some level I felt I had to be as well.

THE CHALLENGE FOR HIV-NEGATIVE GAY MEN

After much thought, many revisions of this article, and several years of therapy I think finding such a fit in the gay community is essential for HIV-negative gay men. While employed at Gay Men's Health Crisis (GMHC), I volunteered to co-facilitate some of the groups for HIV-negative gay men that Steven Ball writes about in this collection. One main theme that ran throughout the groups I facilitated was that men who tested HIV-negative had not had a place to explore what this meant to them as gay men. The group helped me to come to the same realization about my life. One group member dropped out of ACT-UP after being given a bag of pills by a fellow ACT-UPper who could no longer use them. My group member felt he could not tell the guy he was HIV-negative and didn't need the medications. Instead, he retreated into feeling he was lying to people by just being there, pretending to be part of something he wasn't, and that he had no place being there. It was common that the men felt they could not talk to others, especially HIV-positive men, about feeling depressed, overwhelmed, sick, lonely, or unsatisfied with various aspects of their lives. How could their problems compare to the urgency of those experienced by HIV-positive men? The group became a place for all of us, leaders and members, to begin exploring what being gay meant to us, what being gay and HIV-negative meant to us, how AIDS impacted us, and how to try and live through this epidemic.

Several therapists have been theorizing and writing about this merging of "gayness" with AIDS. It is reported commonly that many HIV-negative gay men experience feeling it is only a matter of *when*, not *if*, they will become infected with HIV. I know I've experienced this stressful and disturbing feeling and most group members related this as well. It is further suggested this can unconsciously play a role in engaging in unprotected sex and thus place these men at risk for infection, in a sort of self-fulfilling prophecy. It's not suggested that this is the main reason unsafe sex occurs. In fact, there are many components of normal desires and self-destructive impulses at play that are beyond the scope of this article. The key point is that HIV-negative gay men must find a "fit" in the gay community today and avoid becoming merged or over-identified with the plight of HIV-positive gay men. It is confusing and can be somewhat of a rationalizing process, but is necessary in order to shift the question to *if*, not *when*, I will become infected. I described my experience with this struggle as only an example of one man's attempt to muddle through. I do believe that being able to identify as a gay man without the unconscious joining of HIV into being gay, has had a role in my remaining HIV-negative. The unconscious merger became a conscious, thought-out overlap between HIV and being gay. Instead of feeling like I should be or would become HIV-positive, I worked to help those who were and continued to volunteer in prevention efforts. By doing so, I was working to keep myself HIV-negative, remaining involved in the gay community, and trying to sort out the connection between HIV, gay men, and me. In a sense, I was buying time.

BEING HIV-NEGATIVE AS AN IDENTITY?

At one point during the evolution of the HIV-negative gay men groups, the group leaders were asked to consider the concept of an HIV-negative identity. The idea grew from the understanding that many uninfected men identify with those who are infected. If this was true and if it put men at risk for HIV infection, then encouraging the formation of an identity as HIV-negative might be a way to counter this unconscious process. My co-facilitator and I played with this concept for the ten week run of one of our groups. We attempted to help develop (or elicit) an identity as HIV-negative by responding to group members in ways such as: "How does that affect you as an *HIV-negative* gay man?" or "As *HIV-negative* gay men we . . . " We kept saying the phrase and asking men to view themselves through the lens of being HIV-negative as well as discuss their behavior through this lens. My experience was that this confused the group members. Being HIV-negative was a current condition we all shared, but it did not have the same incorporation into personal identity as seen with HIV-positive men.

I have continuously wrestled with this issue in an attempt to figure out how valid is the concept of an HIV-negative identity. Currently, I feel it makes sense that the men in the group were confused by the forced introjection of this concept. After all, I was. I believe there is a significant difference in incorporating HIV-negative and HIV-positive statuses into identity for gay men. The most glaring difference is that having HIV is a permanent situation. Being HIV-negative is more precarious and not necessarily a stable situation. Prevention has informed us that the only safe sex is non-insertive sex. Condoms can break or be used improperly. The reality is that if you are sexual, you are at risk. The risk may be minimal and reduced to various odds, but any sexually active gay man can tell you that the possibility, however small, is annoyingly present. I will elaborate on this later.

Another difference between being HIV-positive and HIV-negative is that most people do not define themselves by the absence of something. Being HIV-negative means you do not have the virus. It is unusual to form an identity around something one does not have. Being HIV-positive is another story. It involves a viral infection associated with gay sex and activates a political drive for acceptance, against intolerance, and is fueled by its life-threatening potential. These are the things identity politics are all about, taking something society considers "bad" and reclaiming it as "good" and putting it out there for all to see in a new way, with pride and dignity. The HIV-negative person has an absence of HIV. It is a condition but not usually a core identity. An individual's identity is not usually something that can easily be changed. By definition it is part of who you are. Not having HIV does not seem to carry the essential components for such an identity.

When I was approached to write this article, I did not think it would be so hard to write. One reason it has been difficult is that the topic is vague and does not give a starting point. I know David Klotz, the man whose article in this collection is about sero-converting while coordinating an HIV prevention program. In a strange way, I envied his task because he had an event to write about, his sero-conversion and how he reacted to it. Becoming HIV-positive gave him a container from which to explore his situation. I had no such event, nothing specific and tangible, to write about. This strongly parallels the discussion of finding a "fit" in the gay community and developing a gay identity without the need to become infected. My envy of perceiving his task as clearer and more contained eerily parallels the unconscious motivations to become HIV-infected in order to feel a part of the gay community. I do not believe that attempting to achieve or "organize" around an HIV-negative identity is the solution. Rather, an identity formed around being gay that is not so strongly linked to HIV may be more achievable and meaningful.

WHERE'S PREVENTION?

Engaging in and exploring the above concepts cannot occur in many current prevention programs. However, these programs are the majority of services available to HIV-negative gay men. One-shot presentations and half-day workshops cannot meaningfully address such psychological motivations for behavior or provide safe and trusting environments for men to open up to these experiences. Much about HIV and AIDS changes quickly and requires that we constantly stay informed and meet the new challenges. This is easy to see in HIV treatment, but applies equally to HIV prevention efforts. Currently prevention professionals fall into two schools of thought. Ekstrand et al. (1993) and Davies (1993) summarize these polar philosophies as risk elimination versus risk reduction respectively. Ekstrand et al. state "our ultimate goal is to eliminate HIV transmission . . . while we agree that this goal will never be achieved, there is simply no alternative . . . How can we as health educators promote any behaviors or strategies that may expose a person to HIV . . . ?" (p. 281). Davies summarizes "we need to encourage and facilitate the emergent strategies of 'negotiated safety,' rather than condemning them as irresponsible. The implicit goal of eradicating unsafe sex is unrealistic. It is neither a sustainable strategy nor an epidemiological necessity, but rather an unnecessary restriction on desire and action" (p. 280).

SEX AND THE HIV-NEGATIVE GAY MAN

Negotiating sexual activity is complex and HIV has only made it more so. Just what is safer sex for gay men? Is it using a condom for anal intercourse and oral sex? Is it not having anal intercourse? How about having oral sex without a condom, but not to the point of ejaculation in the mouth? These are some commonly voiced plans men use and prevention programs grapple with. Others are not so openly addressed, for example, isn't the risk for infection different for a man getting fucked than for the man fucking? Doesn't oral sex carry the same discrepancy for risk of infection? What are the implications for two HIV-negative gay men? For serodiscordant couples, isn't there a difference in risk and what each can do sexually to the other (for example, can the positive man swallow his negative partner's semen?). How men handle these types of questions, and how prevention professionals assist with these struggles over how to have normal sex in these times, deserves attention. Of the two prevention strategies summarized above, "negotiated safety" attempts to address these types of questions. Negotiated safety is a term researchers coined to describe sexual decision making strategies they identified in a sample of gay men. This is important because the researchers were interested in how gay men incorporated safer sex messages into their daily lives. Gay men got the messages from public campaigns and then began to personally integrate them in ways that were not expected.

ANOTHER PERSONAL STORY

Being involved in HIV prevention as well as a consumer of their efforts, I did not simply adopt the "standard safer sex" message of condoms all the time for oral and anal sex. My decisions about what I would do sexually (including what barriers to use, if any) varied depending upon the situation I was in and numerous other situational aspects. I believe that safer sex is not just a one time decision. Instead, it must be re-made and re-evaluated for every sexual encounter, even if the decision remains consistent.

When I was running safer sex workshops in college, I was careful to be non-judgmental and presented sexual behaviors on a risk spectrum including high, moderate, low, and no risk activities. Having said this, the spectrum was prejudiced towards the message of using condoms 100% of the time as a goal to reach. As my thinking grew more complex, I became less comfortable with our standard message of condoms 100% of the time in order to be safe. My main source of discomfort was my own sexual activities. I was not using condoms all of the time. I didn't feel like what I was doing was wrong, but the discrepancy bothered me. Today, the concept "negotiated safety" describes what I was doing on my own with no guidance. I talked to few people about it and those who I did talk with, spewed back to me the same prevention jargon I gave out in a workshop. It sounded good and clear, but was not my experience of what really happened. As a newly out and sexually active gay man, I wanted to know what it felt like to fuck without a condom, get fucked without a condom, and to taste cum. My then boyfriend was HIV-negative and I was HIV-negative (we had both tested recently), so why should we use condoms? We had talked about sex outside the relationship and agreed if it happened we would tell each other before having sex again. I felt "uneasily comfortable" with this type of sex in my relationships. All of my boyfriends and one night stands started with using condoms. It was after beginning to date that inevitably these discussions and negotiations came up.

I said "uneasily comfortable" because I knew there was always a theoretical or potential risk. Even when I used condoms, there was still the mental jump to worry if a small hole existed, if semen spilled out, or somehow HIV would find its way onto a finger and then into my eye, mouth, or anus. Earlier, I mentioned that the risk for HIV, however small, is always annoyingly present for any sexually active gay man. Accompanying this annoying presence is the equally annoying anxiety it produces. Anxiety has become incorporated into the emotional experience of sex for all gay men. How we deal with it is what varies.

One way I know this is true for me is that I have incorporated HIV testing into my general health care. I do it about once a year because I'm sexually active and even with the precautions I take, it might still be possible to become infected. There are numerous examples of how during and after sexual encounters, the fear (rational or irrational) entered my mind. One example occurred several years ago when I went out dancing in an East Village club and met this guy (I'll call him Vincent) I had once before been introduced to. We cruised each other, met, danced, talked and then we left together. I spent the night with him and our sex included anal sex. He wore a condom, and right when he was coming, the anxiety crept up. On the one hand I was turned on and didn't want him to stop, but I also had flashes of: "should I have him pull out" and "should I make him pull out when I hadn't come yet?" This all happened in seconds and my decision was not to stop because the condom would protect me if he had HIV. He stayed inside of me and pulled out after I came. Less than a week later, my best friend called to tell me Vincent had a boyfriend who was upset because he just found out he was HIV-positive and that Vincent must have been the one who infected him. My friend was calling me for assistance through GMHC, where I was working at the time. My friend did not yet know I had slept with this guy as well. I was taken aback and began to panic. I knew we used condoms and that it did not break, but now knowing he had HIV, the anxiety came back.

The HIV-negative groups gave me an insight into how other gay men incorporated safer sex messages into their sexual lives. The strategies utilized by the men varied and changed as well. Some of the men stopped having sex altogether. Some limited sexual activity to jerk-off clubs. One made a distinct difference between clubs where only jerking off is allowed and those that allowed oral or anal contact. He avoided the latter because he was afraid he would succumb to his desire to have anal sex. Others became serial monogamists and practiced negotiated safety in the way previously described. Some men only practiced anal sex as the inserter, feeling it was low risk for HIV transmission.

What the groups showed me was that when provided with a space in which to develop trust, all of the men admitted to not being able to adjust sexual activity by simply adding condoms into their sexual activity and "eroticizing safer sex." This struck a chord with me as my experience had been exactly the same. Hearing other men share how they incorporated safer sex messages into their lives was professionally helpful because I began to better understand how prevention messages were actualized. Personally, I felt relieved to hear from other men who were in the same struggle. We didn't all deal with it the same way, but it was the same issue.

DATING AN HIV-POSITIVE MAN

My current boyfriend, Michael, is HIV-positive. This is the first relationship I have been in with an HIV-positive man. My decision to leave Sarah Lawrence to work as the personal assistant to Larry came from a confused place in which I felt I needed to experience

AIDS on a personal level to really "get it." It was also a way to feel like a part of the struggle and not just a spectator in the stands, trying to belong. Now I find that my relationship with Michael comes from a more grounded and aware place and has nothing to do with desiring the experience of HIV. In fact, Michael has been up-front about his HIV status and I am "moving" slowly because of it. His good health and remaining asymptomatic for many years has helped me relax into developing a love affair with him.

Knowing he is HIV-positive is very different for me than previous relationships. I have had to re-evaluate my comfort level with previously comfortable sexual acts because I know he has a virus I could get. Together we negotiate the kind of sex we have. It is not as easy and smooth as it sounds. We have done things that later concerned us and I have retested to assure I am still HIV-negative. I find myself often looking for ways to rationalize pushing the limits of what I know is risky. For example, he is testing with an "untraceable" viral load and I have to admit that it often enters my mind as a consideration to add into my "formula" for decision-making. Neither one of us wants me to become infected. We are both well-educated about HIV and yet what we do and would like to do sexually is an on-going discussion in our relationship. What is working for us is that we genuinely care about each other, care about ourselves, and communicate the best we can about our feelings and fears. I am no longer "working" from a place of confusion.

CONCLUSION

Because being HIV-negative does not carry the same personal identification as being HIV-positive, and given the merger of HIV and gay men's identification with the epidemic, it is essential that uninfected men are able to find a fit and a place within the gay community. This fit needs to occur without becoming infected with HIV. Being an HIV-negative gay man is a very difficult position to be in and even more difficult to describe. It does not provide the same type of container as being HIV-positive. This is partly responsible for the phenomenon of many gay men feeling it might be easier to "just become infected and get it over with." These types of exacerbated responses become more common as the epidemic continues. Men are exhausted by having to struggle with what is safe during every sexual encounter. With each arrival of new medications comes an increase in these dangerous thoughts.

HIV has a unique relationship to the gay community. Young gay men, like myself, who come out now must deal with the joining of HIV to "gayness" and the preeminent position HIV has in our newfound community. We need to find places and goals that allow us to grow into gay men outside of HIV, while not ignoring our association to HIV. We may even have to create such places and goals.

In this article I've described how I've stumbled through coming out in the AIDS era remaining HIV-negative. My story is just one of many. Every young gay man has his story. In addition, every HIV-negative gay man, regardless of age, has his unique struggle with remaining negative.

Agencies doing HIV prevention need to create places where HIV-negative gay men can come together to share their struggles and experiences in remaining uninfected. An area that needs more examination is how HIV anxiety has become a part of sex for gay men. This is universally present and is being dealt with on a spectrum from eroticizing to impairing sexual functioning. It is only by eliciting the stories from these men and then building upon their experiences, can HIV prevention professionals create relevant and practical ways to prevent the spread of HIV.

REFERENCES

Davies, P.M. (1993). Safer sex maintenance among gay men: Are we moving in the right direction? *AIDS, 7*(2), 279-280.

Ekstrand, M., Stall, R., Kegeles, S., Hays, R., DeMayo, M., & Coates, T. (1993). Safer sex among gay men: What is the ultimate goal? *AIDS, 7*(2), 281-282.

An AIDS Educator's Seroconversion: Education Is Not Enough

David Klotz

SUMMARY. In March 1994, while working as an educator at a prominent AIDS service organization, I seroconverted after engaging in unprotected sex within a relationship. This article will explore the personal journey of seroconversion as I simultaneously worked in developing programs for helping gay men stay uninfected. Since that time there has been a ground swell of activism around primary prevention for gay men, as well as a movement to explore the psychosocial issues that are the core of sexual risk-taking. Besides discussing what was missing in my education, this article will examine the effects of current prevention services for HIV-negative gay men. *[Article copies available for a fee from The Haworth Document Delivery Service: 1-800-342-9678. E-mail address: getinfo@haworth.com]*

From 1989 to 1996 I worked as an AIDS prevention educator with Gay Men's Health Crisis (GMHC), a large AIDS service organization in New York City. The focus of my work was targeting gay-identified men with behavior change interventions to prevent

David Klotz, PA, is currently Program Coordinator for Community Education in the Office of the Mayor/AIDS Policy Coordination for the City of New York. Correspondence may be sent to: Office of the Mayor/AIDS Policy Coordination, 52 Chambers Street, Room 316, New York, NY 10007.

The author thanks Steven Ball for his support and encouragement.

[Haworth co-indexing entry note]: "An AIDS Educator's Seroconversion: Education Is Not Enough." Klotz, David. Co-published simultaneously in *Journal of Gay & Lesbian Social Services* (The Haworth Press, Inc.) Vol. 8, No. 1, 1998, pp. 13-21; and: *The HIV-Negative Gay Man: Developing Strategies for Survival and Emotional Well-Being* (ed: Steven Ball) The Haworth Press, Inc., 1998, pp. 13-21; and: *The HIV-Negative Gay Man: Developing Strategies for Survival and Emotional Well-Being* (ed: Steven Ball) The Harrington Park Press, an imprint of The Haworth Press, Inc., 1998, pp. 13-21. Single or multiple copies of this article are available for a fee from The Haworth Document Delivery Service [1-800-342-9678, 9:00 a.m. - 5:00 p.m. (EST). E-mail address: getinfo@haworth.com].

13

the further sexual transmission of HIV. Shortly before I started my job, I took the HIV-antibody test for the first time, and the results came back negative. Many of my initial reactions were typical; the ones I remember most are: relief, a sense that I had a new lease on life, and gratitude that I would be one of the survivors. I also realized that my test results had implications for the job I was about to embark on: I was living proof that safer sex worked, a paragon of the success of the type of AIDS prevention education that GMHC had pioneered. Hopefully, I would be able to use myself as a model and transfer some of the successful strategies that had kept me uninfected to my brothers in the gay community.

I continued to test HIV-negative on a regular basis for the next five years. I trusted and believed in condoms and never had unprotected anal intercourse with any of my numerous sexual partners, with the exception of one man with whom I had an intense relationship from 1989-91. We were monogamous, and I was with him when he received his first ever (negative) test result. I had expressed my desire to have unprotected anal intercourse with him if he should test HIV-negative, and after he received his test result, we stopped using condoms. I felt safe with this decision, even though I had been inculcated with the values of my own prevention messages ("use condoms *every* time," etc.). Knowing as much as I did about HIV (I trusted in the accuracy of the antibody test), and being desperately in love with my partner—wanting to experience the intimacy of a barrier-free encounter and trusting him with my life–I had few qualms about not using condoms. With the confidence of my knowledge as an AIDS educator supporting my decision, we enjoyed the intimacy and intensity of latex-free sex until the end of our relationship. My subsequent negative test results confirmed the rightness of my decision, and after becoming single again, I had no difficulty reverting to condom use with new partners, some of them anonymous, some not.

In 1993 I became involved in another relationship with a man who disclosed to me, after some time, that he was HIV-negative. We used condoms for about six months, but as we became closer emotionally we began to push the boundaries of safer sex, negotiating the decision to have anal intercourse without condoms the way most partners do: without words. Finally we ratified with words what our bodies had already done, but the conversation, conducted in the heady afterglow of sex, had lasted only a couple of minutes. It seemed like a reasonable choice–after all, we were both HIV-negative, and although not monogamous, I assumed we were both smart enough to be safe in any encounter outside the relationship. My previous experience with unprotected sex had made me feel safe without the benefit of closely analyzing my choice and its ramifications. In addition, I had been sexually active for so long (since before the beginning of the epidemic), that I had begun to grow complacent about my prospects of getting infected. I just didn't think that it would happen to me, especially since I was armed with the knowledge of safer sex, knowledge which I was paid to impart to others.

In March 1994, two weeks after my partner ejaculated inside me (and not for the first time), I developed a flu-like syndrome, which a friend suspected might be seroconversion illness. At the time, I was enrolled in a pre-vaccine feasibility study of HIV-negative gay men called Project ACHIEVE. The study is an attempt to see what the seroconversion rate of a cohort of sexually active gay men is so that they will have a baseline when they begin clinical trials of preventive vaccines. The men in the study will presumably be among the first to be recruited for trials. I went to Project ACHIEVE for a p-24 antigen test, and to my complete shock (I had thought that I was merely suffering from an ordinary flu) it came back positive. The result was later confirmed with the standard antibody tests. The day after my test result, my partner got tested and his result also came back positive. Since I had tested negative just a month before, and I did not have unprotected sex with anyone else, it was evident that he had infected me.

Numb from the news, I initially felt disassociated from the world around me. I couldn't believe that people's lives could go on as usual while I was in such an acute state of crisis. After this passed, many of the expected reactions followed: sadness, loss, regret, depression, and a great deal of unfocused anger. I was angry at my partner for infecting me, but felt conflicting feelings that I shouldn't direct my anger at him because I don't think he intentionally infected me or withheld information, and because he was simultaneously coping with the difficulties of testing positive, compounded by guilt feelings arising from his having been the source of my infection. It seemed more appropriate under the circumstances to direct the anger at myself: How could *I* of all people, a supposed AIDS prevention expert, have allowed this to happen? Feelings of shame and guilt about my actions, my sexuality and my identity were particularly powerful at this point (although I still had not resolved the troubling feelings of anger that I felt towards my partner).

I have always thought of myself as an extremely sex-positive person who has a very successfully integrated psyche around sexuality, including strongly resolved feelings concerning anal eroticism, which is one of the most difficult psycho-sexual issues for gay men. The anal taboo, which can cause so much dread or shame in gay men, was not an issue for me. Nevertheless, I experienced pangs of guilt, and found myself wishing that I had never had anal intercourse. Although I have long felt, and still believe, that anal intercourse, especially as the receptive partner, is a transforming experience for a man, in the wake of my seroconversion, I found myself ruing that I had ever learned to enjoy it. I felt as if I had committed suicide for a good fuck.

I have always considered my gayness to be a wonderful gift, in spite of the pain, loss, and difficulty involved in claiming a gay identity. Nonetheless, in spite of my radical queer identity and total outward lack of negative ideation around my homosexuality, I found myself needing to consciously fight homophobic feelings that welled up in the wake of my seroconversion. I found myself entertaining thoughts like: "if only I had been straight, then I would have lived a long life," or "the homosexual lifestyle really does lead to illness and death." Luckily, a positive sense of my gay identity was strong enough that these feelings were relatively fleeting and I was able to overcome these ugly persecutions from heterosexual society by consciously reassuring myself that AIDS is a naturally occurring epidemic that has presented a particularly harsh obstacle in the path of sexual liberation, and not a judgment on our "lifestyle." Unfortunately, many people in my position struggle less successfully with the shame and guilt that getting infected engenders and have deep-seated homophobic feelings brought to the surface or reinforced.

My feelings of shame and guilt not only connected to my personal predicament, but also to my strong sense of community and responsibility: somehow, by getting infected I had let down the entire gay community. I had held myself up, both in private and public, as a paragon of how someone could enjoy a healthy sexuality and remain HIV-negative. I had had sex with hundreds of men in a variety of contexts over the years while remaining HIV-negative by simply never getting fucked without a condom. I held up my own example to often incredulous gay men that it was possible to have multiple partners in an urban epicenter and stay healthy. I still believe that this is true and that the particular circumstances of my seroconversion bear this out. Nevertheless, I felt as if I had failed to live up to my own standards, that I had failed to even obey plain common sense. Above all, by becoming another "victim" of the epidemic, I had failed to fulfill the most important part someone can play to ensure the survival of the gay community: to stay healthy and alive.

As my anger abated, my principal feeling in the months after testing HIV-positive was one of loss. I had hoped to live a reasonably long life span, to spend a comfortable middle age traveling, going to cultural events, doing the things I like to do, and not worrying about "settling down" for a while. Now I felt as if my time had been cut short. The future is unknown and unknowable, and it was always a fantasy that I would live to a certain age, but now I'm cognizant of the fact that it is a fantasy. Given the current treatment outlook, and the unlikelihood that I will be hit by a bus or suffer a heart attack (I'm only 32 and in otherwise reasonably good shape), I will probably die of AIDS, which is a horrible way to die (although new advances in treatment are giving me some cause to hope for an extension of my healthy years).

I eventually realized that I had adjusted to this new reality when my depression gradually lifted and I became able to enjoy life again. I've gotten my health care options in place and I have a tremendous amount of support from my extended family of friends. I try to keep in the forefront of my consciousness the attitude that I will enjoy life as fully as possible in whatever time I have, but the reality of HIV, which is very disheartening, is always in the back of my mind. In the past, whenever things were not going as I wanted, I would think to myself that I could have had any of an infinite number of worse fates–the Holocaust is my benchmark for human suffering and my historical consciousness as a Jew is a strong component of my identity—but that is small comfort. I have always tried to keep things in a proper perspective when confronted with tragedy by thinking of how insignificant human life is in the cosmic scheme of things, but that is no comfort when confronted with one's own tragedy; after all, we only have one life, and I felt that I had ruined mine. I had thought I was going to be one of the survivors, that I was home free, but now I'm just going to be one more casualty of this fucking epidemic. As of this writing, my life with HIV has normalized, and I can keep knowledge of it mostly in the back of my mind while I continue *living*, but it is like being under a constant shadow, and I know that life will never be quite the same as it used to be. I'll continue to live, make connections to other people, and do the things that allow me to enjoy life, but now I feel that there will always be a melancholy, a wistfulness, a tinge of sadness and disappointment to everything I do.

After wrestling with my anger and guilt, I determined to refrain from beating myself up for having let this happen. Upon much reflection (and with the help of sympathetic friends), I came to understand that it can be perfectly reasonable to not practice safer sex with a partner. After all, I had done it safely with my earlier partner and it had been a thrilling experience, heightening our physical passion and giving me an intense feeling of trust and openness to him. Unfortunately, with my more recent partner, I made this decision without complete information and without taking the steps that would have ensured our safety. We did not discuss what anal sex without condoms would mean to us, nor did we get tested together and wait six months to be re-tested; we did not talk about our guidelines for honesty and disclosure around unsafe sex outside the relationship. My trust led to a very bad judgment call, but I refuse to feel guilty (or at least struggle not to). The fact is, sex with condoms is *not* normal, and it is reasonable for a couple to want to have unprotected (i.e., normal) sex. There is an ethic in the gay community (partially promulgated by AIDS educators like me) that we have to use condoms *every time we have sex for the rest of our lives.* Try telling that to heterosexual couples and see how many listen! Aside from the obvious implications for trust and intimacy between two people, many HIV-negative gay men are seeking the "protection" of a relationship in order to not have to use condoms. The obvious caveat, which I thought I knew, is that you'd better definitively establish both partners' negative serostatus, and then both have only safer sex when having sex outside the relationship, and be able to discuss any possible unsafe sex with others and its implications.

While I regret not having taken those steps, I partially absolve myself of the blame because I did not have any guidance on the matter. At the time, the issue of couples negotiating unprotected sex was not part of the discourse of either AIDS educators or the gay community. The message I received–and gave out–was "a condom every time." Yet I intuitively knew that this was not a reasonable goal, and that in some situations, gay men will take risks that they view as acceptable and not obey the "100% safe-100% of the time" imperative of safer sex educators. This message makes it exceedingly difficult for people to talk about their true sexual behavior and their risk-taking. The fact that I was the messenger and did not practice what I preached made it that much more difficult for me to talk about it, or to even examine my behavior consciously. Unfortunately for me, this knowledge never materialized in my conscious mind, and I never had a forum to talk about it, or about my desires and the sex I was really having. I felt compelled to present a facade to the world that this safer sex "expert" followed his own rules, that he always used a condom in every circumstance.

Seroconverting has had enormous implications for the work I do and my career. It was incredibly difficult coming into work in the weeks after I tested positive. I wanted to immerse myself in mindless tasks so that I would not have to think about HIV, but it's impossible to escape from it at the offices of GMHC. What made coming to work most painful was that I could not abide the irony that this had happened to *me* of all people, whose job it is to teach safer sex. I thought to myself: What does that say about my abilities as an AIDS educator? How could I expect to save the lives of other gay men if I could not even save my own?

Assuming that these feelings would be common among my colleagues, I found it exceedingly difficult to come out about my status to my co-workers, who knew me as HIV-negative. Although now I'm sure that most would have been understanding, at the time I felt ashamed, and assumed that people would judge me harshly. After an initial urge to withdraw from my work, I eventually resolved that I would continue to work in the field of AIDS education, and try to prevent what happened to me from happening to others. Knowing the bleakness of the prospect for a cure, and the psychological impact of living under a cloud of mortality, my experience has increased my resolve to work harder as a prevention advocate and educator. I also think that I now have a greater understanding of the risks gay men take and the complex feelings that underlie risk-taking behavior.

My situation offers unique possibilities to reach others, but also places some limitations on me in my role as an educator. I continue to experience difficulty in disclosing my serostatus to gay men who attend interventions that I run. I have also disqualified myself from leading GMHC's time-limited support groups for HIV-negative gay men, knowing that I can no longer empathize with the group members, and that the presence of an HIV-positive gay man could inhibit their discussion (as it does in the larger community). I've lived through most of the epidemic as an HIV-negative gay man, and it has been difficult thinking of myself as not able to claim an HIV-negative identity anymore. It's painful to be involved in designing programs for HIV-negative gay men knowing that I can no longer benefit personally from them. When I sat in on the clinical supervision of the HIV-negative gay men who led the groups, I was stricken with a sadness at not being able to take a full role in the process. Hearing the group leaders describe their experience leading the groups and their need to explore parallel process produced a wistfulness that clouded the satisfaction I otherwise derived from the work I had done.

Shortly after the events surrounding my seroconversion, researchers, followed by the media, then educators and activists, started discussing a phenomenon that has come to be called the "second wave": a rising tide of new infections among gay men who were widely believed to have been adequately targeted with HIV prevention services and had successfully changed their behavior. The writings of Walt Odets (1995) began to circulate in the AIDS community and discussion arose about the failures of safer sex education for gay men and the psychological needs of HIV-negative gay men. Phrases like "negotiated safety" (the process of an HIV-negative gay male couple dropping condom use for anal sex) entered the lexicon. A new understanding of prevention issues took hold, focusing on the real risk calculus that HIV-negative gay men make and the incredibly complex psychological factors that impact risk-taking behavior. There had been no open discussion of these things when I made my risk calculus.

At GMHC, I became involved in designing new programs targeted specifically to HIV-negative gay men, I discussed negotiated safety and HIV-negative issues in a weekly advice column I wrote for a local gay publication, and helped design media campaigns that help HIV-negative gay men identify the psychological issues pertinent to identity and risk-taking. I ran workshops where HIV-negative gay men explored their sexual behavior and developed skills to maintain risk-reduction behaviors. And I have been involved in the development of time-limited groups, mentioned above and described later in this collection by Steven Ball, where HIV-negative gay men can delve deeply into issues of identity, loss, life expectations, intimacy, survivor guilt, and the challenge of staying HIV-negative.

Although I can never know for sure, I truly believe that if these discussions had taken place two years before, if there had been a group available to me where I could have explored these feelings, if prevention experts had been talking specifically about the needs of HIV-negative gay men, if the community had been discussing negotiated safety and prevention activism to combat a wave of new infections, then I would probably still be HIV-negative, and I would have a completely different set of life expectations. Finally, I think that I would be engaged at an even deeper level in prevention work to ensure the survival of gay men in this catastrophe: as an HIV-negative gay man working with and connecting to other HIV-negative gay men. Instead, I stand at a remove from the battle, feeling a little like a wounded soldier only able to lend token support from the sidelines.

REFERENCE

Odets, W. (1995). *In the shadow of the epidemic: Being HIV negative in the age of AIDS*. Durham, North Carolina: Duke University Press.

CLINICAL APPROACHES

A Time Limited Group Model
for HIV-Negative Gay Men

Steven Ball

SUMMARY. As AIDS prevention strategies focus more on the psychosocial pressures of gay men who are HIV-negative, group work with this population has proved to be a healing antidote to the ongoing psychological toll of the AIDS pandemic. In an environment in which the link between sex and survival has been turned upside down, groups for these men offer invaluable forums for normalizing fears, clarifying values, disseminating information, and building a community of concern that mitigates overwhelming feelings of loss and isolation that might otherwise lead to self-destructive behaviors. Of particular importance in this model will be stage specific interventions. Recognizing how to utilize an integrative approach within

Steven Ball, MA, MSW, ACSW, is a psychotherapist in private practice in New York City. He is also a consultant at Gay Men's Health Crisis in the Prevention Department. He can be reached at: 626 Washington Street, Apt. 3B, New York, NY 10014.

[Haworth co-indexing entry note]: "A Time Limited Group Model for HIV-Negative Gay Men." Ball, Steven. Co-published simultaneously in *Journal of Gay & Lesbian Social Services* (The Haworth Press, Inc.) Vol. 8, No. 1, 1998, pp. 23-41; and: *The HIV-Negative Gay Man: Developing Strategies for Survival and Emotional Well-Being* (ed: Steven Ball) The Haworth Press, Inc., 1998, pp. 23-41; and: *The HIV-Negative Gay Man: Developing Strategies for Survival and Emotional Well-Being* (ed: Steven Ball) The Harrington Park Press, an imprint of The Haworth Press, Inc., 1998, pp. 23-41. Single or multiple copies of this article are available for a fee from The Haworth Document Delivery Service [1-800-342-9678, 9:00 a.m. - 5:00 p.m. (EST). E-mail address: getinfo@haworth.com].

a time limited framework may give group leaders the best opportunity for exploring the multi-issue concerns related to both staying uninfected and maintaining psychological well-being. *[Article copies available for a fee from The Haworth Document Delivery Service: 1-800-342-9678. E-mail address: getinfo@haworth.com]*

In recent years there has been a growing consensus among AIDS educators: the predominant models of HIV prevention that stress education and information are not stemming the tide of new HIV seroconversion among gay men (Newman, this issue; Odets, 1995). As HIV prevention professionals and psychotherapists struggle with how to serve the array of needs for clients of both serostatuses and varying cultural, social, economic, and ethnic backgrounds, most agree there is an ever-increasing need for specialized interventions at the individual, group, and community levels. Moreover, these interventions must respond not only to the need for general sex education, but also to the psychological fallout of having lived through or been born into over sixteen years of an ongoing biopsychosocial catastrophe.

One prime example of this contextual understanding is expressed in the development and implementation of support groups for gay men who are HIV negative. These groups are proving to be a healing antidote to the ongoing stressors of staying HIV negative. Social group work seems to be a necessary next step in prevention efforts because it can acknowledge and clarify the needs of uninfected gay men while at the same time induce and evoke a sense of community and commonality in gay men who have had little of either.

In an environment in which the link between sex and survival has been turned upside down, groups for HIV-negative gay men offer invaluable forums for normalizing fears, clarifying values, and disseminating information as they mitigate overwhelming feelings of loss and isolation that might otherwise lead to self-destructive behaviors. The positive steps these groups continue to have in fostering a shared vision of community, promoting quality of life and, hopefully, disrupting the process of HIV infection suggest that they may be a helpful model from which to expand our vision of effective prevention strategies into the next century. This essay will describe the ongoing evolution of a ten week support group model developing at New York City's Gay Men's Health Crisis (GMHC) and explore not only its synthesis of theoretical perspectives but the fluid nature by which it continues to incorporate members' experiences in reconfiguring and expanding the group framework.

BACKGROUND

For those of us working in prevention in the early nineties, the ongoing psychological toll of AIDS on the uninfected became like an elephant in our living room: everyone knew it was an issue but no one knew how, or felt entitled, to broach it. No one was prepared for the damage that AIDS would continue to wreak in this decade. Who would have predicted that reactions to HIV testing would divide gay men into positives, those who were infected, and negatives, gay men who escaped the fate of infection but found themselves surrounded by death, illness, uncertainty, sadness, and seemingly endless losses? Nonetheless, openly gay men continued to adapt to their new world and others continued to come out. As all of these men proceeded with their normal human strivings for sexual and relational connection, HIV testing became an important right of passage in gay male development. For many, testing now impacts on every permutation of interpersonal relating, from friendships to early dating to committed partnerships as well as sexual decision making.

In the realm of social services, many HIV negative men have historically felt ignored by the multiplicity of services for HIV positive men, services that did not address negative men's particular social, sexual, or cultural concerns. When uninfected men's complex emotional reactions to the epidemic were not only denied by themselves, but then unconsciously minimized or redefined by their communities as well as social service professionals, obstacles were added to their attaining mental well being and future health (Ball, 1996 a,b). As these men continued to struggle in a world that, however unintentionally, considered their difficulties inconsequential, their growing invisibility triggered old childhood feelings of being an "outsider" and for some, contributed to an acute mental health crisis that often exacerbated behaviors and thought patterns that put them at risk for contracting HIV (Odets, 1995).

Some have argued that in the Eighties, gay men unconsciously colluded with the general public's equation of a gay identity with an AIDS identity (Odets, 1995; Rofes, 1996). The implicit organization of being gay related to HIV, limited the roles of HIV negative men to those of a care giver, mourner/widower or outsider. Some of these men felt that they were not entitled to express their deep fears that they might become infected, or discuss their loneliness or burn-out when so many peers were dying around them. Others reported that they had studiously avoided anything to do with AIDS and were ashamed to tell other gay men that they were afraid or no longer capable of being around illness or death. Many evaded opportunities to share their negative status and sometimes even found themselves tacitly validating the misconceptions of those who assumed they were positive.

Currently, the presenting problems of HIV negative men coming into groups and workshops to address their experience illustrate the legacy of silence around negative serostatus: fear of connecting to other men as friends or lovers; ongoing feelings of anxiety throughout sexual and/or romantic interactions; confusion over all the changing data on HIV; uneasiness telling the truth about their hopes, thoughts and desires; and difficulty maintaining their commitment to safer sex over the long haul.

MEMBER PROFILES

The current climate of change in HIV prevention and the identification of these issues in mainstream media like the *New York Times* (Green, 1996) have begun to publicly validate the issues faced by HIV negative men. After more than a year and a half of offering HIV negative groups at GMHC, what we now encounter from prospective members in the pre-group interview process is an acceptance of the idea that HIV negative gay men *do* have a unique and common set of cultural and psychological issues. They are intrigued by the group flyer that states the groups are about "frank talk about sex, relationships and concerns about your confidence in staying negative" and then reads "the aim of the group is to explore and get support around dealing with these important personal issues." Yet confusion remains regarding how these issues specifically affect their lives and behaviors. It seems most men who get interviewed are experiencing some developmental discomfort as their old beliefs, attitudes, and coping mechanisms are wearing thin.

Among men who came out after the epidemic began, many report that their social, recreational, or sexual patterns are less satisfying and that they no longer have, or never really had, a sense of belonging to any part of the many gay communities. Feeling once again like outsiders actuates a regression, a denial of their pain, that reactivates old developmental issues and childhood wounds. Just as when these men first acknowledged their homosexuality, being HIV negative in the age of AIDS repeats being stuck in a world in which their existence is barely acknowledged and the prospect of their own self acknowledgment means anticipating great losses.

These feelings of isolation and disenfranchisement bare a significant parallel to the pre-coming out stage of being closeted (Coleman, 1982). In order to be adaptive, experiences of "coming out" with one's negative serostatus in a social setting, workshop or group must initiate a process that, like the sexual coming out process, includes new opportunities for connection to others like one's self that redeem, normalize, and depathologize an entrenched sense of difference and isolation. The need for identification is particularly important for prevention professionals to understand when working with HIV negative gay men. Since early in their childhood, most of these men have struggled to find a world that is kind to them, a world that they can trust. They have a sense that they have to grow both internally and interpersonally, but with so many potential role models dead or perhaps emotionally deadened, they don't have a clear vision of what they are growing into. The HIV epidemic has made this struggle much more difficult and has entrenched early conceptions of annihilation.

Men who were "out" pre-AIDS are often exhausted by the subject of AIDS but more importantly, they are also looking for a new sense of belonging and freedom in their lives that can be translated into their sexual and romantic encounters. Many still talk about reconnecting to a valorized past, the Seventies, when they were younger and life was simpler. They want to counteract the learned helplessness that causes many men to retreat into a global ("AIDS affects all I do"), or stable ("it will *always* be this way") vision of their relationships and their immediate community. With members presenting with an impaired sense of future orientation, it becomes necessary to expand their frames of reference away from the tunnel vision of helplessness inherent in safer sex discussions that characterized past prevention workshops and groups, and toward a focus of personal empowerment based on interpersonal relating, exploration, and bringing consciousness not only to particular behaviors but to the particular community in which each man belongs.

AN INTEGRATED MODEL

There came a point where I felt both personally and professionally compelled to create a group intervention that would mitigate the predominant and specious definition of what it meant to be an HIV-negative gay man. Most AIDS service organizations in the early Nineties were still not ready to take on what was seen as a controversial use of limited resources. I, like some other psychotherapists, found it less restrictive and more expedient to set up groups in my private practice setting where I could experiment outside of the confines of the political, administrative, and time restraints of social service organizations.

I continue to offer two long term HIV-negative therapy groups in my private practice which began in 1993. The group psychotherapy/existential framework (Yalom, 1985) used in these groups focuses on interpersonal learning: illuminating members' limited views of themselves and their world as their growing needs for interaction and intimacy help them to focus on improving and expanding their relationships outside of the group. Each weekly meeting seems to provide further evidence for the importance of creating groups that keep members engaged in the long term development of more conscious and personal prevention strategies–strategies that are no longer limited to whether or not to wear a condom, but instead have been refocused on encouraging gay men to support each other for their mutual emotional health and well being.

It has been the effectiveness of these long term groups in helping members grapple with the difficulties of being gay men who are HIV negative that motivated me to start experimenting with a time limited group model. Based on a combination of my private practice groups, as well as experiences with various brief treatment models, I began developing a model that could be integrated into larger prevention programs. The basic assumptions that underlie the use of a brief model are: (1) large numbers of men should have access to the service; (2) multiple groups can provide a link between the members of different groups out into various segments of the gay community, therefore stimulating the environment to further respond to their needs; (3) more volunteer facilitators would be likely to take on group leadership if it had a proscribed impact on their time; and (4) growing numbers of volunteers would reap more benefits for themselves as they continued not only to lead groups, but also to connect with other volunteers.

As of May 1997, GMHC has offered thirty, ten-week groups that have been co-led by various combinations of HIV-negative gay professionals and trained peer facilitators. All of the peer leaders have first participated in the groups and have become an increasingly important resource for leadership. Over three hundred men have taken part in the groups, and each cycle sees more and more men on the waiting list for pre-group interviews. As the model expands to include a couples' group and groups for younger men, the upcoming cycle will offer six simultaneous groups for gay men who are HIV negative.

These mutual aid groups have developed out of a long tradition of social group work that recognizes that participating in a system of people who have common social demands can lead to both socialization and resocialization (Greif & Ephross, 1997). Besides drawing on social group work theory, the groups for gay men who are HIV negative draw on a synthesis of other theoretical perspectives, most notably existential group therapy (Yalom, 1985), gay affirmative self psychology (Cornett, 1995) and narrative therapy (White & Epston, 1990). All of these influences have in common that they are client-centered and supportive, valuing the members' abilities and right to self-determination. Rather than a professional treating a client's pathology, the group leaders are informed participants in a network of reciprocal relationships. This moves away from a more traditional, analytic approach where the facilitator is the professional expert who holds the answer and the group is primarily a context in which to change the individual.

In the GMHC groups, it is acknowledged that since there is only a rudimentary vocabulary for the realities of uninfected men and there are few real experts, group members' self revelations and stories provide the building blocks for expanding and reconfiguring their inner resources. Thus it has been helpful for group leaders not only to understand social group work models but also to use concepts of narrative therapy. Narrative techniques emphasize the telling of personal stories. Yet unlike more traditional therapy that might focus on what went wrong, narrative work searches for the emotional health, the formidable resources that enable people to fight back and survive (White & Epston, 1990). These concepts are particularly beneficial when group members help each other recognize and uncover the extremely varied and unconscious effects of living through fifteen years of a pandemic—effects members may not have previously connected to the impact of HIV. Furthermore, most short term groups tend to focus on one unifying concern, and although these members are united by their desire to stay uninfected, the encouraging of narrative helps many related concerns of loneliness, hopelessness, and uncertainty about the future to surface in the safe container of the "telling" of their experience without the pressure to do something to immediately change the outcome.

This process is particularly beneficial for younger members who may not have experienced the death of someone from AIDS, but whose sexuality and identity are nevertheless infiltrated by the presence of HIV. An example of such helpful story telling happened in a second group when one young man, in an attempt to tell why he valued the group, told of watching one of the first network television dramas about AIDS, "An Early Frost," in his parents' living room at age fourteen. Even though he did not yet consciously identify as gay, he so related to the main characters that he thought it inevitable he would die of AIDS once reaching adulthood. When the group leader asked for analogous stories, the members shared similar stories of first hearing or being impacted by AIDS. By the telling of members' stories, there emerged a collective acknowledgment of how HIV/AIDS had and is affecting dating and hope about being in an ongoing relationship, as well as other core life choices.

As members begin to identify with each others' struggles, they hear their own experiences reflected back to them in a myriad of different group interactions and stories. Through externalization, a central intervention strategy in narrative therapy that defines the problem as external to the individual, members are able to recognize and acknowledge the confusing and oppressive impact of AIDS phobia and homophobia, both external and internal. The struggle is no longer a strictly personal, internal one rooted in the past but instead it is an external and current battle against the communal tragedy of living in the era of AIDS. The articulation of hard-earned heroism can open the door to visions of the future and become the foundation for new life stories that evoke members' speculations about what kind of futures they can have if they continue to see themselves as strong, competent, and supported.

SELF-DISCLOSURE

Self-disclosing is an important and difficult concern for the leaders throughout the life of the group. Often the leaders struggle with how much to share of their related stories if they believe it will further the process of the group or jump start the group and more quickly build cohesion. Until recently, the group leaders have been encouraged, in their weekly group supervision which meets in a parallel process throughout the ten weeks of the groups, to explore disclosing their serostatus from the outset of the first group by employing the term "we" when making initial interventions about the group's purpose.

Just as out gay therapists may serve as positive role models for expanding self-expectations of gay clients, role modeling by HIV-negative men seen as informed professionals or peers can provide group members with a sense of permission to claim and explore the distinct experience of living as HIV-negative gay men. Leaders have shared instances from their life stories to deepen and clarify the group process (Glassman & Frederick, this volume).

It has become increasingly clear that the groups are not about exploring and embracing a stable HIV-negative identity. Therefore, the newest cycle of groups at GMHC will include men who do *not* know their HIV status, as well as those who do. Sometimes, even men who have tested still feel that they are unsure of their current status based on their uncertainty about the test or their latest sexual activities or psychological stressors. In a drop-in group for gay men who are HIV negative which I co-lead, the inclusion of men who have not tested has helped, by comparison, the men who *do* know their HIV status to further understand what it means to them to remain uninfected. Reciprocally, it has helped those who have never been tested to hear from others who have been through similar struggles to clarify and make conscious their decision regarding whether to test. In groups of members who have undetermined HIV status or mixed serostatus, the issue of self-disclosure and HIV concordance/discordance becomes much more difficult to resolve (Ball, 1996 a,b). Since self-revelation could become a hindrance to exploration of the differences among members, group leaders in these revised ten week groups will not disclose their HIV status as readily in the early stages of group as freely as in a non-mixed group.

It is important to recognize that the use of peers to co-lead the groups provides invaluable opportunities for group members to interact with others like themselves. The peer volunteers include a mix of mental health professionals and lay volunteers all of whom have participated in the ten week groups as members and received training in HIV prevention and group facilitation. Not surprisingly, many of the lay peer facilitators, more readily than the professionals, use their seroconcordance to build group cohesion by offering examples from their own lives to help legitimize members' feelings and concerns. This not only continues the therapeutic work for the peers themselves but also has often compelled the professionals to explore how they might more effectively use themselves and their life experiences in service of group interaction.

MEMBER SELECTION

The importance of the process of selecting and preparing the members for group cannot be emphasized enough, and is one of many areas that warrants further study and experimentation. As in most groups, the face to face pre-group interview is not only an assessment, but more importantly an orientation process that includes an agreement from the potential member to work cooperatively within the short term format. The interviewer asks about an individual's interpersonal patterns and roles in "natural" groups in their lives to date, including their family of origin and family of friends. If they are in acute risk, including an eruption of psychotic process, suicidality, homicidality, or extraordinary, severe anxiety, or in a situational crisis such as the recent death of a loved one, they are referred to more appropriate interventions. Some are referred to short term counseling, while others may be referred to a less intensive one time or three session group.

Men who are referred out during the pre-group interview are encouraged to return to the group in the future, after more immediate clinical concerns have been addressed. Members are not screened out for using alcohol or drugs outside of the group, as this often becomes a topic for interaction in group. In accordance with a harm reduction model, the group can serve the important function of pre-contemplation and contemplation, essential steps on the road to responsible drug use or recovery. In several pre-group interviews, however, it has become apparent to the client that his substance use is of greater concern than his negative status and he has then been told of the Substance Use, Counseling and Education Department at GMHC, where he may explore more specific issues about his substance use. In the case of acute mourning, some clients have attended a bereavement group before entering the ten week groups.

Group construction includes the traditional complexity of composing a group with a balance between homogeneous and heterogeneous elements. Group composition requires some homogeneity of ego strengths and experience to insure that no member becomes a scapegoat or outsider. For instance, a member at the very beginning of his coming out process would probably be better served in a coming out group or the "New Generation" ten week group which is described in the flyer for "guys who initially started thinking about sex after the early Eighties, when HIV and AIDS became a part of everyday lives."

In the groups at GMHC, as we continue to experiment with group composition, we are presently working to balance different ages, experiences, relationship status, and developmental levels within most of the groups. It is true that heterogeneous factors such as age and differences in experience initially can create a baseline tension.

However, when correctly facilitated, these differences can be used in the service of building interpersonal curiosity which accelerates the pace of the group.

Although an acknowledgment of the similarities of experience of being HIV-negative defines the beginning efforts of group cohesion, the members inevitably end the ten weeks with a sensitivity to each member's right to be different. Certain themes related to individuality, separateness and autonomy, clearly lacking in the general safer sex guidelines of past prevention campaigns, are played out and examined in the group, as a result of the differences among group participants. The interpersonal and experiential variety of participants parallels membership within a community, and as a result, the groups more effectively reflect their outside environments and foster intergenerational cross talk. Along with the leaders, the wide variety of members provides poignant opportunities for role modeling and mentoring for men of different ages and backgrounds.

STAGES OF GROUP DEVELOPMENT

Of particular importance in this developing model are stage specific interventions that utilize a developmental perspective of group work. Roy MacKenzie (1990), a leader in the subject of time limited group psychotherapy, describes a six-part system that incorporates the developmental stages of a group into a therapeutic "road map" that has proved helpful in predicting behaviors for these groups. The themes that emerge that are specific to the experience of being gay men who are HIV negative are integrated into the group leader's understanding of group development in order to help him to recognize predictable group behaviors during specific stages. This framework not only helps the leaders to foster a sense of progress through the ten week experience but also prevents the group from getting derailed by issues unrelated to the particular stage.

During the first stage of engagement or affiliation, members generally speak consciously about how to stay uninfected. They begin to talk about the sex they are having; they compare notes about whether or not they are dating or in relationship with HIV positive men, and they confess some of their anxieties and anger at not having clear answers about how to negotiate their sex and romantic lives. Underneath these conscious interactions, the latent content revealed in this early stage is often a desire for a more heartfelt sense of *belonging* to the group, which functions as a microcosm of the gay community. Often members express this dynamic more by how they interact than by the content of their verbal expressions. Leaders often attempt to help the men to verbalize these concerns about affiliation by asking the members to fantasize how they hope this group and these particular men could be helpful.

In the first session, the leaders are active in providing structure and often ask members to share the goals that they began to formulate in the pre-group interview. They clarify the group's overarching purpose as a safe place where members not only share each others' personal accounts of living as urban gay men, but also focus on interpersonal learning that will help them feel more connected to their world outside of the group. Toward the middle of the first session, the ten members break into pairs where each one interviews the other for five minutes and gathers information that includes a glimpse of each person's past, who they are in the present, and future hopes as it relates to participation in this group. Members are then re-introduced by their partner to the group. This is one of the very few structured exercises performed in every group's process because it is a proven ice breaker. It helps evoke commonalities and differences by enabling the men to make some introductory self statements within a contained, safe framework while encouraging meaningful interpersonal communication.

Leaders are encouraged throughout to bring new ideas into the group system and to share their effectiveness in the weekly supervision group. Many group leaders give a homework assignment that asks the members to continually notice how the groups affect their daily lives. One set of group leaders experimented with having the members filling out a weekly card where they reflected on the group during the week and focused on issues and concerns they had difficulty sharing in group. At the beginning of the next group, members handed the cards back to the leaders. The leaders read the cards after group and usually responded in writing by encouraging the member to bring up their concerns in group. These weekly cards helped leaders monitor individual concerns that might not be appropriate to the agreed upon goals of the group and helped to monitor potential group drop outs. Other leaders have written a weekly letter to the group in an effort to enhance continuity, their witnessing of the group life, and the bridging of the group into their outside world.

In the first three meetings, men over thirty-five often tend to talk about themselves in connection to those who are positive or have AIDS, minimizing their own needs. It seems as if it is safer to talk about grieving and loss because these ideas are more socially acceptable than talking about their desire to stay negative or make meaningful connections. This reflects an implicit value code among gay men regarding who is and who is not entitled to have a psychological reaction to the epidemic. Many gay men who are HIV negative have felt that they are permitted only one reaction, that of grief related to the immediate loss of a close personal relationship when someone dies of AIDS. Many have felt that any other reaction was gratuitous and self involved–a narcissistic response. Throughout the group process, this legacy becomes apparent and acknowledged. Only then do the members recognize that grief is affecting their lives in much more complex and individual ways than they had previously believed. The group begins the process of shedding the social stigma of being uninfected and gay. By talking about loss in general the men claim a right to a more truthful experience, where multiple losses are acknowledged as well as the loss of disease-free sexuality, the loss of free and uncomplicated interpersonal connections, the loss of a sense of a pleasurable future, and the loss of an idealized gay community.

The general anxiety of the early stage of groups is reframed for the members as a first date. This metaphor of dating is often invoked throughout the group process to mirror the developmental stages in building a relationship and to normalize the members' conflicts and anxieties about getting closer to each other versus running away from the intensity of the connection.

By the third session, most groups begin to move into the middle phase of differentiation, where members often wrestle with the discomfort of getting closer to each other and their desire for and fear of connection. The manifest content presents as discussions of difficulties with dating and sex and the intersection of these two areas. This stage is exemplified by the recognition of individual uniqueness that includes physical, sexual, and spiritual differences among members. The group has moved out of childhood, so to speak, and is moving into adolescence, where sub-groups emerge and conflict and power struggles start to get explored. Sex becomes an even more pervasive topic. Although anxiety remains high in this stage, it is acknowledged more readily. Interestingly, confrontation frequently focuses on how the different members choose to interact socially and sexually with HIV positive men. Contrary to the initial group focus on HIV positive men that comes from a place of self-effacement, when the subject arises in the middle phase, discussion starts to emanate from a place of growing self-awareness and entitlement. As the facilitator reinforces productive interactions that focus not only on content, but also on how members are dealing with each other interpersonally, these men begin to realize how their feelings and emotions affect their behaviors both within and outside of group.

When men begin to explore ambivalence regarding safer sex practices, it often signals the beginning of the third phase of individuation. Safety has been tentatively established and members begin to disclose their personal concerns. In one group, a battle developed between what got labeled as the "sex positive" men versus the "sex police." The sex positive men seem to claim their sexual expression over the fear of being in a culture hyper-aware of HIV and the men they designated the "police" were men who were seen as making negative judgment about those men who wanted to keep having sex or unprotected sex without making any "real sacrifices."

Even the most complaisant members sometimes seem to get pulled into such conflictual discussions when they begin to express frustration about continuing to hold their interpersonal and erotic needs in abeyance. Most groups find themselves locked in an ongoing debate over the safety of oral sex. In one group, some members believed that the leaders were privileged to the latest safer sex information and were intentionally withholding answers from the group. The fact was that the leaders were in the same psychological place as the members; they did not have the answers. After the leaders explored the source of these feelings and fantasies, they then attempted to highlight the common difficulty of not having the magical answer to safer sexual encounters. When one of the leaders revealed his struggle and his thought process while making sexual decisions, he set off a process of self disclosing that helped members to consciously realize that they have to struggle with finding out what level of risk is individually acceptable for them.

As the members continue to acknowledge their mutual conflicts, they move tentatively into the stage of intimacy. As the group becomes more consciously familial, the content of the group sessions concerns interpersonal acceptance, rejection, and realistic expectations of each member for the others. If the group works harmoniously, this stage quickly intertwines with the phase of mutuality in which members experience how moments of altruism and reciprocity can exist while still holding on to their own distinctive needs, wants, and desires. In one group, a poignant moment occurred in the ninth session when members started fantasizing about what it would be like if they all lived together, going into great detail about how it would be to come home to one another, even discussing whether or not the leader would be there. They joked about how each one would take care of the others, and how it would feel to be surrounded by men with whom they could share their true feelings about the day, about last night's date or sex, and about their relationships. It is important to note that for some of the men this is a different orientation to caring from the "care-giver" role with which they entered the group. These men still doubted that they could create this sense of closeness and trust with friends outside of the group—but the success of the group was to know it was possible.

In the final phase of termination, the members investigate ways to continue to appreciate and enjoy their lives as they attempt to value and hold on to the lessons of communication and validation experienced in group, while gathering their inner resources to deal with the confusion that is still to come as they live as gay men amidst the complexities of a world infected by HIV. As is the case in all brief groups, the final phase of separation and termination concludes with many experiencing a desire for the group to continue in order to avoid confronting the loss of connection. Throughout the group process, the methodical countdown to termination enables the men to use the group as an emotional laboratory in which they can explore and experiment with issues of anticipatory loss similar to those that many are experiencing and might experience in their daily relationships. As members process the loss of the group, a final task for the leaders is to assist members in identifying both triggers for feelings of isolation and newly understood sources of validation and support. Leaders encourage members to speak openly about their fears of returning to a place of constriction and alienation once the group is terminated.

One favorite closing exercise is to have the men write a letter to themselves that they would like to receive one month after their group terminates which reminds them of their group experience and helps them stay connected to whatever they found most helpful. Co-leaders collect these letters in the final group and do mail them one month later. This can help integrate the story of the group into the narrative reality of members' lives. Many men express a desire for another group experience, and some have gone on to other groups. Some are training to become peer facilitators in future groups. For many of these HIV-negative men, the ten week support group offered the first safe place where they could openly explore their emotional response to the AIDS epidemic, while gaining a sense of membership, acceptance, and approval in a community setting. Keeping these men healthy and HIV-negative requires helping them find hope for their future, confidence in their abilities to make significant, meaningful connections with one another, and faith that they can find ways to appreciate life even while they gather the inner resources to deal with the pain and loss that is still to come.

FUTURE DIRECTIONS

In a group with so many converging issues, ten weeks of interaction can only point the way to a modification of thinking and relating regarding the many issues raised during the course of the group process. Based on several rounds of focus groups held after the ten week cycles, the groups seem to have the most positive outcomes when the style of leadership is active, caring, and supportive as it maintains a "here and now" focus. While the response from the focus groups suggests that these ten week groups have proven important and effective resources for many participants, they are by no means a panacea to seroconversion. Currently, the research and evaluation department at GMHC is doing more scientific inquiry into the outcomes of these ten week groups versus a one time discussion group or workshop type intervention.

There are clearly clients and groups of individuals that will not respond to the therapeutic guidelines examined in this article. The groups described consisted mostly of urban white men, between twenty-one and sixty-three years old who for the most part identified as gay. The guidelines described are not intended as a rigid "cookbook" but are best viewed as a summary of pooled experience that worked well with this population at this time in our collective history. Using the clinical framework articulated in this article while at the same time remaining flexible and creative when it comes to outreach, orientation, and expectations, may make this model accessible to many other groups of marginalized men.

The time has come to expand the place of groups in prevention campaigns and make them available to those who do not have access to the social services they both need and deserve. Hopefully, this group model will spark new ideas and strategies that will strengthen the capacity and motivation of all HIV-negative gay men to believe in a future for all gay men, regardless of HIV serostatus, with an integrated understanding of how HIV is continually affecting their lives and relationships.

REFERENCES

Ball, S. (1996a). Serostatus and counseling. *Focus: A Guide to AIDS Research and Counseling, 11*(8), 1-4.

Ball, S. (1996b). HIV-Negative gay men: Individual and community social service needs. In M. Shernoff (Ed.), *Human services for gay people* (pp. 25-40). Binghamton, NY: The Haworth Press, Inc.

Coleman, E. (1982). The developmental stages of the coming out process. In J.C. Gonsiorek (Ed.), *Homosexuality and psychotherapy: A practitioner's handbook of affirmative models* (pp. 31-430). New York: The Haworth Press, Inc.

Cornett, C. (1995). *Reclaiming the authentic self: Dynamic psychotherapy with gay men.* Northvale, New Jersey: Jason Aronson Inc.

Green, J. (1996, September 15). Just say no? *New York Times Magazine*, 38-45.

Greif, G. & Ephross, P. (1997). *Group work with populations at risk*. New York: Oxford University Press.

MacKenzie, K.R. (1990). *Introduction to time-limited group psychotherapy*. Washington, DC: American Psychiatric Press.

Odets, W. (1995). *In the shadow of the epidemic: Being HIV-negative in the age of AIDS*. Durham, North Carolina: Duke University Press.

Rofes, E. (1996). *Reviving the tribe*. Binghamton, NY: The Harrington Park Press.

White, M., & Epston, D. (1990). *Narrative means to therapeutic ends*. New York: W. W. Norton.

Yalom, I. D. (1985). *The theory and practice of group psychotherapy* (Third Edition). New York: Basic Books.

When Seronegative Gay Male Therapists Work with Seronegative Gay Male Clients: Countertransference Issues in Time-Limited Group Psychotherapy

Noah S. Glassman
Ronald J. Frederick

SUMMARY. With the growing awareness of the impact of AIDS on seronegative gay men comes a need for clinicians to respond effectively to this population's unique issues. Seronegative gay male therapists, however, often face the same unaddressed issues shared by their clients. Therapy groups focusing on the concerns of uninfected gay men are relatively new, and therefore few of the seronegative gay male therapists facilitating these groups have had a forum for examining their own experiences as uninfected survivors of the epidemic. Consequently, these clinicians must navigate various countertransference feelings (e.g., overidentification with clients) as they interpret group issues that match their own concerns (e.g., serocon-

---

Noah Glassman, PhD, is a post-doctoral fellow sponsored by the National Institute of Mental Health in the Psychology Department at New York University. Ronald Frederick, PhD, is a clinical psychologist at St. Luke's Roosevelt Hospital Center, HIV/AIDS Center and has a private practice in New York City.

Address correspondence to Dr. Glassman at NYU Psychology Department, 6 Washington Place, 7th floor, New York City, NY 10003 (E-mail: noah@ psych. nyu.edu).

[Haworth co-indexing entry note]: "When Seronegative Gay Male Therapists Work with Seronegative Gay Male Clients: Countertransference Issues in Time-Limited Group Psychotherapy." Glassman, Noah S. and Ronald J. Frederick. Co-published simultaneously in *Journal of Gay & Lesbian Social Services* (The Haworth Press, Inc.) Vol. 8, No. 1, 1998, pp. 43-59; and: *The HIV-Negative Gay Man: Developing Strategies for Survival and Emotional Well-Being* (ed: Steven Ball) The Haworth Press, Inc., 1998, pp. 43-59; and: *The HIV-Negative Gay Man: Developing Strategies for Survival and Emotional Well-Being* (ed: Steven Ball) The Harrington Park Press, an imprint of The Haworth Press, Inc., 1998, pp. 43-59. Single or multiple copies of this article are available for a fee from The Haworth Document Delivery Service [1-800-342-9678, 9:00 a.m. - 5:00 p.m. (EST). E-mail address: getinfo@haworth.com].

version fears, survivor guilt). Using their personal experiences as co-therapists of time-limited groups for seronegative gay men, the authors outline identification and group-process issues, and offer strategies for managing and using countertransference reactions to benefit clients in this work. *[Article copies available for a fee from The Haworth Document Delivery Service: 1-800-342-9678. E-mail address: getinfo@haworth.com]*

As detailed by others in this volume and elsewhere (Ball, 1996; Johnston, 1995; Odets, 1994, 1995; Rofes, 1996), seronegative gay men experience their own set of unique issues as a result of living in the middle of the AIDS epidemic. These men may be caregivers for ailing lovers, they may have had many losses to AIDS, they may be surrounded by HIV-positive friends, and they may feel alienated from a gay community where gay identity sometimes seems equated with being HIV-positive. When they test negative, their anxieties about seroconversion, and the impact HIV has on their lives, does not end. Trying to remain negative can feel like walking a tightrope–a feeling made even more palpable by a seronegative test result. Moreover, testing negative can trigger its own concerns, anxieties, and questions. For example: Can I trust my test results? Can I tell my HIV-positive friends about my serostatus? How can I talk to my HIV-positive friends about my difficulty with safer sex when their *own* problems seem so much more pressing and serious? How much longer can I stay negative? What kind of safer sex guidelines can I truly live with? and How can I allow myself to feel close and intimate with another man when I'm constantly obsessing about HIV?

At a time when infection rates among young gay men are increasing (e.g., Stall et al., 1992), these questions, which are only a handful of those facing uninfected gay men, highlight the urgent need for clinicians to respond effectively to this population's mental health issues. Because psychotherapy groups focusing on the concerns of uninfected gay men are relatively new (Ball, 1996; Johnston, 1995), few of the seronegative therapists facilitating these groups have yet had their own forum for examining their experiences as uninfected survivors of the epidemic. Consequently, these clinicians are left to navigate unexplored aspects of their own experience as they interpret group issues that match their own concerns.

They are susceptible to becoming overwhelmed by their own feelings about the epidemic's effect on them, and they may experience intense overidentification with their clients' worries. In this chapter, we outline the types of countertransference reactions that can arise in doing this work by examining our own personal responses to facilitating time-limited therapy groups for HIV-negative gay men. More specifically, we discuss the impact of unexplored aspects of one's experience on clinical work and illustrate ways in which therapists can make clinical use of their reactions to enhance group process. Although we describe countertransference in the context of group therapy in particular, much of what we discuss is also broadly applicable to individual therapy/counseling situations. Furthermore, the topics covered are relevant to clinicians as well as peer counselors/facilitators, both of whom play important roles in many HIV/ AIDS prevention programs.

COUNTERTRANSFERENCE: GOOD OR BAD?

Historically, countertransference has had various definitions, with infrequent agreement about its meaning and usefulness as a therapeutic tool (e.g., Greenson, 1974; Reich, 1951; see also Laplanche & Pontalis, 1973; Tower, 1956). In the classical view (Freud, 1963), countertransference stemmed from the therapist's own psychopathology and referred to a therapist's "irrational" or "distorted" reactions to a client's transference. From this perspective, countertransference was considered a problematic aspect of treatment to be analyzed and dispensed with tidily in the therapist's own personal therapy (Grossman, 1965). Although later developments in the conceptualization of countertransference asserted its value in psychotherapy when it is acknowledged and skillfully used by the therapist (e.g., Little, 1951; Racker, 1957; Winnicott, 1949), countertransference continues to have negative connotations to the extent that it is seen as reflecting the therapist's "weakness," "errors," or "blind spots" (e.g., Cohen & Farrell, 1984; Langs, 1982).

For the purposes of the present discussion, we describe countertransference in terms of the therapist's capacity for understanding the client's experience by *identifying with* the client's position in the world (i.e., "concordant" countertransference; see Racker, 1957).[1] In this vein, we consider countertransference as an expectable, normal, and even essential aspect of therapy that contributes to empathic understanding, while it also acknowledges the therapist as an individual with real, human reactions to others. Countertransference is not something to be avoided or swept under the rug once it is understood. Rather, we view countertransference reactions as ongoing aspects of the therapeutic work that we are continually processing. Moreover, we endorse the use of countertransference as a therapeutic resource for furthering clients' benefits from treatment. It is from this perspective that we examine our experiences of facilitating group therapy for uninfected gay men.

FIRST REACTIONS:
WHAT DO SERONEGATIVE GAY MEN
HAVE TO COMPLAIN ABOUT?

Having therapy groups for HIV-negative gay men is a controversial issue that has met with considerable resistance by several voices in the gay community (Ball, 1996; see also Rofes, 1996). In describing our countertransference reactions to facilitating these groups, it is necessary to start at the beginning, that is, with our reactions to the very idea of uninfected gay men having their own issues and needs.

When we were first approached about running groups for HIV-negative men, we wondered: "Why do healthy uninfected men need a forum for discussion? Why waste resources on something like that when there are so many infected and sick members of our community to attend to?" Even thinking of doing these therapy groups made us feel that we were betraying friends, acquaintances, and clients who were either HIV-positive or who had died from AIDS. We worried that it would appear that we were forsaking the needs of seropositive gay men by focusing on the seemingly illuso-

---

1. Although there are obviously other types of countertransference identifications, such as identifying with the reactions and feelings of important people from the client's past or present life (i.e., "complementary" countertransference; Racker, 1957), addressing these aspects of the therapist's experience are beyond the scope of the current discussion.

ry concerns of "neurotic" seronegative gay men. Telling our HIV-positive friends that we were considering facilitating such therapy groups would certainly be insulting to them, or so we were convinced. We were afraid that it would look as though we were forming our own clique or club for uninfected gay men.

Our attitudes began to shift, however, after we read the writings of Walt Odets (1994, 1995). As HIV-negative gay men, we had many HIV-related issues and dilemmas in our lives that were as yet completely unaddressed, and moreover, that were exacerbated by messages within our own community. For instance, safer-sex messages (e.g., "100% safe, 100% of the time"), failed to take into account what made sense for our individual lives by treating sex without condoms under any circumstance as something inherently "wrong." Such messages imply that our sexual desires, even before we have acted on them, are pathological and dangerous and that we should not even give voice to these desires, much less give in to them. We had unknowingly introjected these messages wholesale. Consequently, as William Johnston (1995) explained, "virtual HIV" had intruded upon our sexual and romantic relationships. That is, even though we were not HIV-positive, the specter of the virus was affecting us nonetheless in terms of our feelings about sex, intimacy, the future, and ourselves. We did not yet have the language, however, to talk about the ways that we were being affected by HIV and AIDS.

Our feelings about being seronegative in the middle of the epidemic remained untapped because we did not notice them. Even though we were uninfected, we never felt secure in our HIV-negative serostatus, and were often consumed with thoughts and worries about becoming infected. While witnessing so many people being ravaged by AIDS, we could not feel happy or satisfied in our lives. Moreover, we found it increasingly difficult to even imagine our futures, to think about growing older, feeling convinced on some level that we would not live long lives. Our early ignorance, and perhaps outright denial, is surprising to us now when in retrospect it is quite apparent how ubiquitous HIV was and is in our lives.

GROUP THERAPY AS PREVENTION TECHNIQUE

A growing awareness of the concerns of HIV-negative gay men (e.g., Fisher, 1996; Green, 1996), coupled with rising infection rates, has led to new prevention efforts. Therapy groups for seronegative gay men, conducted from various models (e.g., see Ball in this volume; Johnston, 1995), have begun around the country–all with the goal of keeping these men uninfected by providing a forum for addressing their experiences of being HIV-negative in the middle of an epidemic. The groups we facilitate are time-limited, lasting 10 weeks, and typically consist of approximately 10 clients and 2 facilitators. From the outset, we introduce ourselves to the group as seronegative gay men in an effort to provide a safe environment in which the members will feel free to express feelings and opinions that may, in other contexts, seem "politically incorrect" or "insensitive" to those who are HIV-positive. Although withholding the therapists' serostatus from the group may also have potential therapeutic benefits–for example, allowing the group to speculate about the status of the facilitators can bring into the transference members' conflicting emotions about their seropositive friends and lovers–we place an emphasis on creating safety in the group environment, given the time-limited nature of the treatment. Furthermore, having therapists self-identify as HIV-negative gay men who are not "in the closet" about their serostatus can provide important modeling for the group.

Men in the group are given the opportunity to voice worries they feel inhibited about expressing with others, and in turn their experiences are often validated by other group members. They also discuss the different meanings various sexual acts have for them, and come to realize that people in the group have different values. Reflecting on these values eventually informs decisions that they make about what levels of risk they are willing to have in their sex lives. Moreover, essential to group psychotherapy is the acknowledgment of common ground and similarities among group members, as well as the recognition and acceptance of the differences among them. These aspects of the group dynamic mirror the basic processes of merger, separation/individuation, and integration that are crucial elements of all close and important interpersonal relationships (Alonso & Rutan, 1984, 1996; Bion, 1959).

In addition, part of our work with seronegative gay men involves fostering an "HIV-negative identity" (Odets, 1995), which we conceptualize within a developmental framework similar to the coming out process. Group members must first "come out" as HIV-negative gay men before eventually integrating this part of themselves into their overall identity—much in the way that adolescents struggle to identify and explore different parts of who they are before arriving at a more fluid integration of the different aspects of themselves. Importantly, the group eventually moves into discussions of intimacy needs in relationships within and outside of the group. Ultimately, we hope to foster connections between group members, to cultivate an orientation toward the future, and, as a result, to motivate group members to stay alive and uninfected.

As white, uninfected gay male therapists who came out in the age of AIDS, there are many issues we will not be able to speak to here. For example, there are issues unique to the experiences of African-American, Asian-American, and Latino uninfected gay men, as well as to gay men who were out before the onset of the epidemic, that we will not address because discussing countertransference requires us to speak from our *own* experience, and to do otherwise might seem presumptuous. However, racial and ethnocultural issues are obviously important and need to be kept in mind when doing this work. Having made these caveats, we now turn to what happens when seronegative gay male therapists are faced with the same unaddressed issues shared by their uninfected clients in group therapy.

GROUP FACILITATORS OR GROUP MEMBERS?

As several of us in a supervision group were about to start our first therapy groups for HIV-negative gay men, we all expressed our envy of the men in our groups. We realized that even though we were about to facilitate these groups, we had never had a forum for talking with other gay men about our *own* experiences of being HIV-negative. We had many unprocessed feelings about being uninfected in the middle of the epidemic, and we envied the opportunity our group members had for beginning to process these feelings. As a result, when our group began, there was a strong pull to join the group; we wanted to become group members (Alonso & Rutan, 1996).

Having these feelings engendered a conflict within us about how much self-disclosure, as therapists, was appropriate. Of course, self-disclosure is determined in part by one's therapy orientation and personality style, but overidentification with our clients around issues we had barely begun to explore in ourselves added another level of complexity to making therapeutic decisions. On the one hand, the pull to join the group made sharing our personal experiences very tempting. After all, when group members talked about their obsessive worrying over potential infection from past sexual acts, or when they described their difficulty with being convinced that they did, indeed, have futures, we were having those feelings as well. On the other hand, we also became alarmed, at times, by the extent to which we identified with group members and the feelings they expressed. Moreover, we were discovering new feelings and reactions along with the group. Group discussion sometimes hit too close to issues that we had not yet processed ourselves, and as we realized this we felt constricted and reluctant to share our experiences and reactions with the group. This raised an essential question: What kinds of self-disclosures would be for our own personal benefit, and what kinds of disclosures would benefit the group?

In grappling with this dilemma, we realized that in-depth discussion with each other about our reactions to the group was crucial. Each week we described to each other the ways in which the anxieties and concerns expressed in the group mirrored our own. Having group supervision was also important in giving us space to begin to recognize our own issues as we tried to help the group deal with similar ones. Once we were secure in having time to work through our reactions to the epidemic, our seronegative status, and the group, we felt better able to recognize and work with the parallel issues raised by group members. Processing our reactions with each other freed us to make decisions about discussing our own experiences and reactions with the group in ways that would facilitate the group process (see also Isay, 1996 for more on the relationship between self-disclosure and countertransference in gay clinicians).

Using questions from our own lives, for example, facilitated group discussion of topics that members seemed reluctant to articulate. In a session in which sexual practices had become the focus of discussion, we provocatively asked the group if there is ever a time when unprotected sex is "OK." In raising this question—which was one evoked, in part, by our own experiences—we hoped to communicate to the group that it was all right to talk about impulses, feelings, and behaviors that may seem forbidden in other contexts. One group member responded, "I feel like we've all been giving the 'A+' answers, talking about how we all have safer sex, but when I was with my last boyfriend, we decided to have sex without condoms because we were both negative and monogamous. It feels like nobody ever talks about that." This admission eventually led to a much broader and more open discussion of the emotional meanings people give to various sexual behaviors, moral judgments associated with these behaviors, and the psychological impact of safer-sex guidelines. Thus, reflecting on our own HIV-related conflicts helped us to identify unspoken issues in the group and enabled us to provoke deeper interactions about these issues among group members.

SERONEGATIVE, BUT FOR HOW LONG?

A common feeling among HIV-negative gay men is their sense that their negative status is an ephemeral condition. Many men doubt the permanence or the reality of their negative status. For instance, one group member emphatically expressed his fear that he would wake up one morning having spontaneously seroconverted during the night. The predominant perception among the men in our groups is that they are more likely to become positive—like everyone else in their lives, or so it seems—than remain negative. A common sentiment that we hear in our groups is, "I'm negative . . . for now."

Because we may have similar feelings about our own negative status, our own anxiety can become triggered when group members begin to express such feelings of inevitability. The group process often begins with a release of pent-up fears about seroconversion that terrorize many HIV-negative gay men. This release, which can sometimes be like an explosion, is prompted by finally having a space to discuss that which has gone unspoken for so long. Many men are isolated with these fears as they feel unable to discuss them with others who may see such worries as trivial and unimportant. In the early stages of the group, men bond through the sharing and unburdening of these fears with other HIV-negative men. Group members allow their anxiety, which is often overwhelming for them, to come to the fore and be validated by the group. During this time, the group leader is extremely susceptible to overidentification with patients and their fears if he has not yet begun to work through his own anxieties.

Moreover, as we have seen in the groups we run, it is not uncommon for HIV fears to surface at critical points in gay men's lives, such as at the beginning of new challenges and endeavors—especially when embracing future-oriented goals (e.g., career enhancement, relationship commitment, etc.). For instance, one of us found himself in an especially difficult position during the early stages of our first group. Shortly before starting this group, he had begun a post-doctoral fellowship in HIV/AIDS at a metropolitan hospital. Surrounded in the hospital by people sick with AIDS, he started to have a great deal of anxiety about his own HIV status and was quite convinced that he indeed was infected, even though his sexual history indicated a low probability of this being the case. He was tested before the group began, but he did not receive the results until two weeks later. At our first session, he wondered if he should even be in the group, if he might, in fact, be an impostor. How would the group members respond to his leaving the group if he tested positive? What would this mean to them? What would it mean to him and to us? His results came back negative before the second group, but his renewed negative status was tenuous, at first. He began to examine more deeply his fears of being infected and grew alongside the group members in his understanding of his own issues related to his negative status.

When therapists begin to address and make sense of these issues in themselves, they are then able to understand where HIV-related concerns come from in group members—i.e., when they are irrational, and when they are not. We say "*begin* to address" because we do not think it is entirely necessary to have completely processed these and related issues before doing this kind of work; rather it seems sufficient for the therapist to have begun this process, and to continue it while working with this population. At the same time, hearing the thoughts and feelings of group members can help put our own feelings into perspective and, as a consequence, enable us to be in a better position to help our clients. With an understanding of one's own issues, the therapist can begin to help clients move past their anxiety to come to understand that feelings of inevitably becoming infected can arise out of a mixture of irrational and perfectly rational ideas. One can then begin to clarify the confused thoughts, beliefs, and emotions that become entangled with feelings about having HIV. Often beneath issues related to HIV are feelings about being gay (e.g., internalized homophobia; Frederick, 1996) and issues that are of a more dynamic nature. Once one moves past the initial anxiety, making sense of the underlying factors becomes possible.

For instance, one group member, Mike, spent several sessions talking at length about his intense fear of seroconverting and how this fear seemed to rule his life. In one session he announced that he had had a "scare" the night before that he very much needed to discuss. He described a scenario in which he was having anonymous sex with another man in a sex club and accidentally cut himself. He turned his body away from his sex partner so that he would not be exposed to this stranger's semen. In telling his story, Mike wanted the group to reassure him that he had not put himself at risk and to help him put an end to his worries—which they tried to do. When we first started running these groups, we might have become sidetracked by Mike's fears as his story might have tapped into our own strong anxieties about our sexual behavior. We may have felt the same impulse to try to reassure him that he tried to take precautions to protect himself. Instead, however, we wondered why this man, who professed to be so worried about getting infected, was putting himself at risk not only physically, but emotionally as well by frequently allowing himself to be in situations that served to perpetuate a cycle of obsessive worrying. Having started the process of reflecting on our own anxieties regarding our sexual behavior and HIV status, we did not feel as vulnerable to Mike's anxiety, and were thus in a better position to challenge him to begin to examine and understand his own behavior and the internal forces that compelled him to put himself at risk.

THE "WORRIED WELL" TAKE A BACK SEAT

Our struggle to address our own needs as HIV-negative gay men played out in the groups in several other ways, as well. For example, we initially felt, as the group members did, that our anxieties and concerns as uninfected men were trivial and inconsequential in the face of so many sick and dying friends and lovers. Weren't we the "worried well" who had no business whining or complaining in the middle of an epidemic? As group facilitators, we were forced to confront these feelings as we tried to address the needs of a group member, Sam, whose lover was very sick with AIDS. At first, we colluded with the rest of the group in believing that Sam's issues were far more important, more serious, and more pressing than anyone else's. The group process seemed to stall as we became preoccupied with wanting to ensure that Sam was getting enough support and attention in the group. Moreover, none of the group members were talking about their reactions to Sam and his pressing concerns. He seemed to remain outside of the group and was increasingly withdrawn. We began to worry that he would have been better off in another type of group, but we knew that he had already been through a group for caregivers of people with AIDS, and that he was looking for something more.

Eventually, as we recognized that we had our *own* difficulty with feeling entitled to voice our needs and concerns as HIV-negative gay men, we realized that Sam was not allowing himself to have *his* own needs. We realized that he had much to gain by owning an HIV-negative identity, by joining with other group members around this identity, and through this process, eventually being able to envision a future for himself–something that was very difficult for him to do when he first joined the group. Coming to terms with our own reluctance to feel entitled to have needs freed us to encourage the group to talk about their reactions to Sam. Although they expressed their fears that he was judging their HIV-related anxieties as "stupid" or "trivial," the group also let Sam know that they wanted to feel closer to him and to see more of him. Sam's attitude toward the group and toward his own life seemed to begin to change as a result. He surprised us in a subsequent session when he spontaneously engaged other group members in a lively conversation about his strong feelings about HIV-prevention work and his ideas for helping adolescents remain uninfected. We had never seen him so related to others, so full of affect, and so oriented toward his own future. Even though he was in the process of beginning to mourn the loss of his lover, he seemed to begin to find ways to remain invested in his own life. As therapists, we felt that becoming more in touch with our own difficulty with feeling entitled to our own needs ultimately enabled us to work more effectively with the group by feeling more confident about its usefulness and its importance.

GRAY AREAS IN THE BEDROOM

In facilitating these groups, we also had to reflect upon our own ambivalence and anxiety about adhering to safer-sex guidelines. As therapists, we felt a strong pull from the group to resolve the ambiguity of some of these guidelines. The group members wanted clear, black-and-white rules that would help alleviate their anxieties about how to have safer sex while still enjoying sex. They felt plagued by guilt and worry if they strayed from established guidelines. In particular, they worried about having oral sex without condoms, and in their urgent need to have these worries allayed, they even imagined that we were withholding from them the latest, conclusive, research findings about the risks of oral sex. The anxieties expressed by the group triggered our *own* anxieties about the ambiguity we are forced to live with in *our* sex lives. When one group member described how eating Cap 'N Crunch cereal gave him a panic attack because it tore his gums after giving a blow job, we joined the rest of the group in laughing nervously. The story was comical, but it was also serious. As much as we wanted to alleviate the groups' anxiety, as well as our own, we recognized that we had no real black-and-white answers to offer.

Our impulse to want to provide magical solutions for the groups' worries came, in part, from our own need to have these answers. But ultimately, we knew that we had to learn to tolerate some ambiguity, some scary gray areas, in our own sex lives. Our task then, was to try to help the group to tolerate this ambiguity as well by having each of them reflect upon their own feelings and values, and by having them ask themselves what kinds of risks, if any, they were willing to live with in their sex lives. For some of them, it was the first time they truly allowed themselves to connect to how they *felt* about safer sex, and it was the first time they thought carefully about what kinds of guidelines would make sense for them as individuals.

BARRIERS TO INTIMACY

While the groups we run are organized around attempting to address the concerns of HIV-negative gay men, we believe that a major thrust of the groups is to help HIV-negative gay men relate to each other in a manner that is more emotionally intimate than they are typically accustomed to doing. Our belief is that when we as HIV-negative gay men become better able to relate with other gay men and to connect in a more intimately satisfying way, we will come to better value our lives and ourselves and, consequently, be more committed to staying uninfected.

There are many barriers to intimacy that are especially common and formidable in the relationships of gay men (e.g., Shernoff, 1996). HIV is one of them. Many men are afraid of getting close to others as they believe, on some level, that the relationship will not last, or that they will be abandoned as a consequence of AIDS. These issues of abandonment become intensified in the time-limited group situation where the men are very much aware of the clock ticking away and termination drawing near. As one of our group members expressed, "Why should I get close to people in the group when the group is going to end and everyone will go away and I will be alone?" Of course, HIV is not the only reason for difficulties with intimacy, but it sometimes becomes the container for a host of other issues, and as such it is often more readily apparent in the group context.

What is of interest here to us as therapists is the challenge we face in facilitating closeness among group members when we ourselves may be grappling with our own issues of closeness. The group context itself, that is, being in a group of several gay men, may foster the therapist's own issues with intimacy to come to the fore. In running the groups, we became, and continue to become, even more aware of our own struggles with intimacy, wondering how we can be of help to these men when we ourselves are also struggling with being intimate in our own lives and relationships. What has been helpful to both of us in doing this work has been an awareness of our own conflicts, knowing that they are there, and then remaining open to learning from the men in the group about ourselves as we help them to identify and understand their own issues. For instance, it became apparent to us in the seventh or eighth session of one of our groups that our reluctance to talk with each other between sessions about the group allowed us, on one level, to avoid dealing with the ending of the group, and more personally, to avoid having to experience the loss of the group ourselves. When we acknowledged this conflict, we more easily understood our group members' own ambivalences about intimacy, and their reluctance to begin to grapple with the loss in closeness that the groups' ending signaled. With an awareness of one's own issues with closeness, the therapist can then help group members struggle with, and begin to work through, intimacy issues and termination in an adaptive way by making space for often avoided feelings.

SUGGESTIONS FOR MANAGING COUNTERTRANSFERENCE IN GROUP WORK WITH HIV-NEGATIVE GAY MEN

In conclusion, there are several things that one can do as a therapist working with HIV-negative gay men to help understand or work through one's own HIV-related concerns which, in turn, will ultimately help to facilitate therapeutic work: (1) Reading the emerging literature on the issues facing seronegative gay men can help clinicians recognize their own unexplored or unrecognized reactions to living in the age of HIV/AIDS. Acknowledging the impact of the epidemic on our own lives was an important first step in helping us to work therapeutically with the men in our groups. (2) What we have also found extremely beneficial is spending time together immediately before and after the groups to discuss the internal responses and reactions we experience during sessions. Through these discussions, or process sessions, we not only came to better understand the group, but also ourselves. (3) In addition, we felt more empowered as gay men as we began to accept being seronegative as part of our own identity. Beginning to come out as an HIV-negative gay man fosters the process of accepting this aspect of one's identity and facilitates therapeutic work with clients. (4) Group supervision has several functions. It not only provides one with necessary supervision, but it also serves as a forum in which therapists can talk about their own HIV-related concerns, get support from their colleagues, feel less isolated with their own issues, and, as a result, move forward in their acceptance of their own HIV-negative identity. Having our needs addressed in this critical way ultimately frees us to be better able to meet the needs of our HIV-negative gay male clients and, in doing so, helps us to be better, more effective therapists.

REFERENCES

Alonso, A., & Rutan, J. S. (1984). The impact of object relations theory on psychodynamic group therapy. *American Journal of Psychiatry, 141,* 2-6.

Alonso, A., & Rutan, J. S. (1996). Separation and individuation in the group leader. *International Journal of Group Psychotherapy, 46,* 149-162.

Ball, S. (1996). HIV negative gay men: Individual and community social service needs. *Journal of Gay & Lesbian Social Services, 4,* 25-40.

Bion, W. R. (1959). *Experiences in groups.* New York: Basic Books.

Cohen, F., & Farrell, D. (1984). Models of the mind. In H. H. Goldman (Ed.), *Review of general psychiatry* (pp. 23-36). Los Altos, CA: Lange Medical Publications.

Fisher, I. (1996, July 14). Support groups for HIV-negative gay men. *The New York Times,* pp. 25-26.

Frederick, R. J. (1996, August). *Internalized homophobia: Theoretical and clinical implications.* Paper presented at the 104th meeting of the American Psychological Association, Toronto, Ontario, Canada.

Freud, S. (1963). Further recommendations in the technique of psychoanalysis: Observations on transference-love. In P. Rieff (Ed.), *Freud: Therapy and technique* (pp. 167-180). New York: Collier Books. (Original work published 1915).

Green, J. (1996, September 15). Flirting with suicide. *The New York Times Magazine,* pp. 39-45, 54-55, 84-85.

Greenson, R. R. (1974). Loving, hating, and indifference toward the patient. *International Review of Psychoanalysis, 1,* 259-266.

Grossman, C. M. (1965). Transference, countertransference, and being in love. *Psychoanalytic Quarterly, 34,* 249-256.

Isay, R. A. (1996). *Becoming gay: The journey to self-acceptance.* New York: Pantheon.

Johnston, W. I. (1995). *HIV-negative: How the uninfected are affected by AIDS.* New York: Plenum.

Langs, R. J. (1982). Countertransference and the process of cure. In S. Slipp (Ed.), *Curative factors in dynamic psychotherapy* (pp. 127-152). New York: McGraw-Hill.

Laplanche, J., & Pontalis, J. -B. (1973). *The language of psycho-analysis.* New York: Norton.

Little, M. (1951). Countertransference and the patient's response to it. *International Journal of Psychoanalysis, 32,* 32-40.

Odets, W. (1994). AIDS education and harm reduction for gay men: Psychological approaches for the 21st century. *AIDS & Public Policy Journal, 9,* 1-18.

Odets, W. (1995). *In the shadow of the epidemic: Being HIV-negative in the age of AIDS.* Durham, NC: Duke University.

Racker, H. (1957). The meanings and uses of countertransference. *Psychoanalytic Quarterly, 26,* 303-357.

Reich, A. (1951). On counter-transference. *International Journal of Psychoanalysis, 32,* 25-31.

Rofes, E. (1996). *Reviving the tribe: Regenerating gay men's sexuality and culture in the ongoing epidemic.* Binghamton, NY: The Haworth Press, Inc.

Shernoff, M. (1996, January). Chronically single. *In the Family,* 16-21.

Stall, R., Barrett, D., Bye, L., Catania, J., Frutchey, C., Henne, J., Lemp, G., & Paul, J. (1992). A comparison of younger and older gay men's HIV risk-taking behaviors: The communication technologies 1992 cross-sectional survey. *Journal of Acquired Immune Deficiency Syndrome, 5,* 682-687.

Tower, L. E. (1956). Countertransference. *Journal of the American Psychoanalytic Association, 4,* 224-255.

Winnicott, D. (1949). Hate in the countertransference. *International Journal of Psychoanalysis, 30,* 69-75.

The Challenge of Staying HIV-Negative for Latin American Immigrants

Alex Carballo-Diéguez

SUMMARY. Homophobia, fueled by the anti-homosexual rhetoric of the Catholic church, is rampant in most Latin American countries. This conceptual paper postulates that, in the same way that ethnic culture is deeply entrenched in Latin American groups living in the U.S., transgression of social rules, as a gay-survival strategy, is an intrinsic part of Latin American gay men's psychological functioning. Many of these men, who experience moving to the U.S. as a personal Stonewall Rebellion, are subsequently reluctant to accept restrictions on their sexual expression. Although they are aware of the HIV risks presented by unsafe sex, they equate safer-sex guidelines to the moral and social taboos that they circumvented. In this context, HIV-negative gay men feel that they can get away with still one more instance of unprotected sex. This paper highlights the need for critical thinking about internalized homophobia and transgression survival mechanisms as prerequisites to self-empowerment and HIV-prevention behavior among men who have sex with men of Latin American ancestry. Individual and group psychotherapy and community level political activism may contribute to this end. *[Article copies available for a fee from The Haworth Document Delivery Service: 1-800-342-9678. E-mail address: getinfo@haworth.com]*

Alex Carballo-Diéguez, PhD, is a research scientist at the HIV Center for Clinical and Behavioral Studies at the New York State Psychiatric Institute and Colombia University. Correspondence may be sent to: HIV Center for Clinical and Behavioral Studies, New York State Psychiatric Institute and Columbia University, 722 West 168th Street, New York, NY 10032.

[Haworth co-indexing entry note]: "The Challenge of Staying HIV-Negative for Latin American Immigrants." Carballo-Diéguez, Alex. Co-published simultaneously in *Journal of Gay & Lesbian Social Services* (The Haworth Press, Inc.) Vol. 8, No. 1, 1998, pp. 61-82; and: *The HIV-Negative Gay Man: Developing Strategies for Survival and Emotional Well-Being* (ed: Steven Ball) The Haworth Press, Inc., 1998, pp. 61-82; and: *The HIV-Negative Gay Man: Developing Strategies for Survival and Emotional Well-Being* (ed: Steven Ball) The Harrington Park Press, an imprint of The Haworth Press, Inc., 1998, pp. 61-82. Single or multiple copies of this article are available for a fee from The Haworth Document Delivery Service [1-800-342-9678, 9:00 a.m. - 5:00 p.m. (EST). E-mail address: getinfo@haworth.com].

The boy he'd engendered was an aberration, someone my adolescent father couldn't define or recognize as his own. He looked at me and hated himself because he'd created a monster. Worse yet: a *mariquita*.[1] (Muñoz, 1996)

How do we help HIV-negative men who have sex with men (MSM) of Latin American ancestry to stay uninfected? In New York City, one of the world's epicenters of the AIDS epidemic, surveillance reports indicate that while the incidence of AIDS among European American MSM decreased from 68% before 1985 to 44% in 1994, MSM of Latin American descent experienced an increase from 14% to 26% (New York City Department of Health, 1995). This increase has been attributed to the insufficient or inappropriate allocation of funds for the prevention of AIDS among minorities; to the endemic problems of poverty, racism, and discrimination that affect them; and to lack of cultural sensitivity in prevention campaigns (Culturelinc Corporation, 1991; de la Cancela, 1989). This paper focuses on some aspects of Latin American culture vis á vis homosexuality that should be taken into account in HIV prevention, both at individual and community levels. Only after the reader reflects on the importance of gender roles and homophobia in Latin America, the harmful role of the Catholic church, the harassment and extortion that MSM experience in the hands of the police, the prejudice against homosexuality that mental health practitioners have, and the insufficient organization of the gay community will he or she understand the oppressive climate in which homosexuals develop in Latin America, the transgressive survival mechanisms they resort to, and the role these mechanisms play in unsafe sex.

GENDER ROLES AND HOMOPHOBIA

In contrast to sex as a biological reality, gender can be described as a socio-cultural construction by which certain human characteristics are said to be masculine whereas others are said to be feminine. Strict gender-role differentiation characterizes Latin American soci-

---

1. Faggot, effeminate man.

eties. Octavio Paz, the Nobel prize-winning Mexican writer, describes this in his book *Labyrinth of Solitude* (1993). Paz highlights the Mexican's association of manliness with introversion, impenetrability, secretiveness, mistrust, hostility, toughness, stoicism, and formality. Femininity, a complex issue in Paz's words, is related to creation, tenderness, and resilience to suffering, but also to passivity, sin, vulnerability, and openness to intrusion. Although men from other Latin American regions, particularly those from the Caribbean, may be less introverted than Mexican men, their societies still put a strong emphasis in distinguishing *macho* roles from those of women (de la Cancela, 1986; Ramírez, 1993).

In this universe of dichotomous gender roles, a man who conforms to the macho ideal does not necessarily lose his social standing for having sex with another man, whereas a man "who acts like a woman" is considered inferior regardless of his actual sexual behavior. Studies of MSM conducted in Brazil (Fry, 1984-85; Parker, 1986), Mexico (Carrier, 1977; 1995), Costa Rica (Schifter-Sikora, 1989), Nicaragua (Lancaster, 1988), and Peru (Cáceres & Rosasco, 1993), among others, ratify this observation. In his autobiographical book *Before the Night Falls* Reynaldo Arenas (1994), describing the events that preceded the Mariel boat lift from Cuba, emphasizes the importance ascribed to gender roles in relation to homosexuality.

> Since the order of the day was to allow all undesirables to go, and in that category homosexuals were in the first place, a large number of gays were able to leave [Cuba] in 1980. . . . At the police station they asked me if I was a homosexual and I said yes; then they asked me if I was active or passive, and I took the precaution of saying that I was passive. A friend of mine who said he played the active role was not allowed to leave. He had told the truth, but the Cuban government did not look upon those who took the active male role as real homosexuals. (p. 281)

Although men's manly behavior is expected to flow naturally from their anatomical destiny, it also needs grooming by exposure to other men. Fathers, who are considered responsible for instilling manhood in their male offspring (Lumsden, 1991), are particularly concerned with having macho behaving sons (Ramírez, 1993). A son who is less than optimally masculine casts doubts on the masculinity of his father. Therefore, fathers frequently warn their offspring against the wickedness of effeminacy and make derogatory comments about *maricones* (queers). A recent article in a Dominican publication (Sandoval, 1995) states that in the Dominican Republic it is common to hear fathers state that they prefer to have a son who is a thief or a drug user rather than a homosexual. Quoting Dr. Gómez Montero, a psychologist, the article states:

> The everyday Dominican family sees homosexuals as a threat to virtue, morality, *buenas costumbres* [proper behavior], and the reputation of the linage. . . . The parents of a homosexual feel that they are victims of a terrible punishment, and their reaction to their offspring's coming out is often scare and total rejection. Most parents see homosexuals as perverts, ill people who can infect those in the household. Usually, once they are found out, homosexuals are expelled from their homes and ignored by siblings, in-laws, grandparents and uncles who do not dare discuss the issue in public.

A Cuban man, who participated in one of the studies I conducted in New York (Carballo-Diéguez, 1992) candidly described his father's behavior the day he left the island.

> I consider my father a square person. His fingers are this thick from operating farm machines. He never spoke much at home. He had always thrown in my face that I was a little strange, and that I did not like women. But he did not use the word queer. On that May 11, Mothers' Day, when the police came to look for me, I realized he loved me. He loved me as a son; he just did not want a homosexual son. I saw my father crying for the first time. He took me on a motorcycle to Las Cuatro Ruedas [a detention center close to the Mariel harbor]. That day he even gave me money, which I had to throw away later because they told me that [the police] would take all our money and our jewelry.

E. Bossio, Director of the Lima Homosexual Movement, Peru's only gay rights organization, was quoted in the *Chicago Tribune*

(Marx, 1992) as saying: "Most gays are still in the closet because the social pressure is incredible. I know lesbians beaten by their fathers when they tell them they're gay. I've been kicked by my neighbors."

Given the strong gender-role distinctions and homophobic attitudes described, it is understandable that young men who start to experience attraction to other males feel completely counter normative, are afraid of others finding out their inclination, and consequently try to hide it. In some cases the strategy works, and for many years the homosexual youngster can live a life with the outward appearance of heterosexuality. The advantage of this façade is that he may face less harassment than if his sexual orientation were obvious. However, "passing" does not free the homosexual from experiencing the social demands to conform to the heterosexual ideal, and he is continuously under pressure to date girls, to commit to a woman in marriage, and to procreate. Although young men who "pass" may appear to have an easier time dealing with social demands, they only internalize the struggle and become extremely conscious of all that is at stake if their cover-up is revealed.

Other boys are more obvious in their expression of homosexuality. Those who are effeminate will probably be subject to harassment from peers and adults and most likely receive no support in developing a positive sexual identity. In many cases, these youngsters will be targeted by other males for rape. An effeminate boy is seen in Latin America as a damaged, weak being. A man who sexually abuses an effeminate boy may not consider himself to be engaging in homosexual behavior: rather, he is teaching the young queer a lesson on how a man is supposed to act.

In our study of Puerto Rican men, one third of the participants reported having had their initial sexual experience before age 13 with a partner at least four years their senior. Half of these respondents felt physically or psychologically hurt during the experience, but very few disclosed it to their families. Except for rare cases, those who disclosed the abuse were told not to mention it to outsiders so as not to bring dishonor to the family and themselves (Carballo-Diéguez & Dolezal, 1995).

Those who do not pass for straight have a hard time during their childhood and adolescence, which occasionally makes it impossible for them to finish their studies or achieve other goals and may even lead them to suicide. However, they may also learn early in life about homophobic harassment and may develop ways to cope with it. These men are less likely as adults to be closeted, to get married, or to live double lives. They may be in contact with their inner wishes, be able to express themselves, and to varying degrees let their inclination be known to the people around them, achieving at a younger age a more genuine life style than their closeted peers.

THE CATHOLIC CHURCH

The Catholic church was present in the Americas since the early days of colonization through missionaries who sought to "convert the infidel." Recruitment and induction into Catholicism was done with disregard for local beliefs and habits, with many natives being enslaved or killed in the name of religion. Sexual practices were observed with curiosity, and overt homosexual interactions were deemed unacceptable and punishable (Anabiarte & Lorenzo, 1979).

Catholicism intertwined its power with that of local authorities. This is clearly depicted in the urban plan of most Latin American cities which consists of a central plaza flanked by the buildings of the civilian authority (City Hall, governor or President's home) and the clerical authority (church or cathedral). Prelates were and still are regularly present in official ceremonies, and Catholicism is *de facto* the religion of the state. A citizen may not be candidate for president in many Latin American countries if he or she is not Catholic. Many special benefits are offered to the Church. In Argentina, for example, bishops receive a government stipend equal to the salary of a supreme court justice; the state provides the Church with radio and television stations; and half of the schools are Catholic and receive public funds. Public-school teaching is also subject to the influence of the Church exerted through its infiltration in the government and its education ministries.

In most Latin American countries, the government discourse is often indistinguishable from that of the Catholic church, especially when it concerns homosexuality. On September 24, 1994, the *Washington Post* (Escobar, 1994) reported that, in his weekly television program in Argentina, Cardinal Antonio Quarracino, "known to have the ear of President Carlos Menem," said that gays and lesbians should be sent to what he called a "type of separate country" where they could form their own laws. This, the Cardinal said, would "clean an ignoble stain from the face of society." Quarracino is one of two cardinals in Argentina, the archbishop of Buenos Aires, and the president of the Bishops' Conference.

In other Latin American countries, the Catholic Church had similar homophobic pronouncements. Sandoval (1995) states that in the Dominican Republic the Catholic Church, which does not give communion to active homosexuals, preaches that an important number of men and women present instinctual homosexual tendencies, which constitute for them a real challenge. [The church] considers that homosexuals are called to chastity so that by self-control and the training of their inner freedom they can approach Christian perfection (p. 11).

In Mexico, Archbishop Quintero Arce, a Roman Catholic primate for the northern state of Sonora, called "aberrant" an international meeting of gays and lesbians in Acapulco, stating that it "lowered the morals of the Mexican people" ("Mexican archbishop," 1991). The Catholic church also allied itself with political movements like the Pro-Vida group in Mexico, and exploited the issue of AIDS and safer-sex education in terms of the preservation of "traditional family values" and procreative sex (Lumdsen, 1991).

It is remarkable that a church that blocks the access of women to positions of power, that forbids its male ministers from marrying women, that favors male clergy living in collective quarters and until recently had them wear long black dresses—covered with layers of embroideries for celebrations—would attack homosexuality.

One may think that the Catholic church in the U.S. is equally homophobic and that other denominations also show intolerance of gays and lesbians. The big difference between the U.S. and Latin America in this respect is the lack of religious pluralism found in the latter and the overwhelming majority of Catholicism. This generates a lack of questioning and an acceptance of Catholic dogmas as facts of life. Youngsters who experience homosexual feelings cannot but feel that it is a sin even to entertain same-sex fantasies. It is not a battle between the self and the environment, but rather an inner battle between feelings and a monolithic moral consciousness that represses them.

POLICE HARASSMENT AND EXTORTION

The police and the armed forces are other societal institutions responsible for the spread of homophobia in Latin America. According to Marx (1992):

> In Latin America, military regimes that governed during most of the last half-century either passed laws that outlawed homosexuality or made it difficult for homosexuals to act openly by allowing police to detain them for violating vague laws that prohibit everything from "offending public morality" to having "immoral purposes."

The *modus operandi* of the police is similar across Latin America: Someone suspected of being homosexual is approached by policemen, either in uniform or in civilian clothes, and is threatened with exposure to family members or work mates as well as imprisonment. If the victim offers to pay a ransom, he is generally allowed to go although at times he needs to engage in sex with the "authority." Some homosexuals report beatings and rape in the hands of the police.

Police harassment is vividly portrayed in the voice of a 19 year old transvestite prostitute in Mexico:

> *Lo único malo de este negocio es el acoso de los patrulleros, unos perros que nos exigen dinero para dejarnos trabajar. A veces, cuando no traemos lana porque todavía no ha caído ningún cliente, se agandallan y nos quieren coger gratis. Nos tratan muy mal, nos insultan, nos manosean y nos bajan de putos mamadores. He sabido de tres o cuatro casos de compas a los que de hecho han violado arriba de las camionetas y a quienes después tiran a mitad de la calle, todos magullados, con la ropa en desorden o rota, sin lana, sin zapatos, despeinados o sin peluca. Son unos salvajes pero hasta ahora no hemos podido hacer nada para quitárnoslos de encima y evi-*

*tar sus extorsiones, sus desmanes y su violencia. Nos conside-
ran peor que a putas.*

[The only bad thing about this job is the patrols' harassment, these dogs who demand money to let us work. Sometimes, when we don't have cash because we have not had a
client, they get cocky and want to fuck us for free. They treat
us very badly, they insult us, they feel us, and treat us as
sucking queers. I know about three or four companions who
have been raped in the patrol cars and afterwards have been
thrown in the middle of the street, bruised, with their clothes
messed up or torn, no money, no shoes, disheveled or wigless.
They are savages, but thus far we have been unable to do
anything to get them off our backs and avoid their extortions,
their excess, their violence. They treat us worse than whores.]
(Guillén, 1994)

A Colombian man who participated in one of our studies stated:

*Si lo veían salir de un bar de esos o si Ud. de pronto lucía un
poco [afeminado], pues tenía que huirle a la policía porque en
una o en otra forma le sacaban dinero a Ud.. Eso sucedía con
mucha frecuencia, el chantaje. A mi nunca me sacaron dinero.
Pero amanecí muchas veces en una estación de policía. Siete u
ocho veces. No me sentía muy seguro en la calle. Es parte de
la vida, quizás, en mi país. Lo único que me afectó es que el no
confiar [en] la credibilidad en la policía y quizás en las insti-
tuciones.*

[If they saw you leaving one of those bars or if you looked
somewhat (effeminate), you had to flee from the police because in one way or another they would get money from you.
Blackmail was very frequent. They never got money from me,
but sunrise found me many times at the police station. Seven
or eight times. I did not feel too secure in the streets. It's part
of life in my country. It made me distrust the credibility of the
police and, maybe, of any institution.]

Another Colombian man I interviewed in 1995 reported the en-
trapment techniques used by policemen in movie houses.

It was five years ago. In Bogotá, I used to go to the Faenza theater, which is not gay. . . . Policemen in civilian clothes go there *a chantajearlo a uno* [to blackmail people]. They come and sit by your side, let you touch them, go out with you, and then they threaten you, they ask you for money, they rob you of your watch. If you don't give them money, they take you to the precinct. One time, they took me to a police station at 10:00 p.m. and they held me there till 4:00 p.m. the next day without food and without a chance to sleep. . . . Here, in New York, I would call 911, but there you can do nothing. The system does not protect you. Each one is on his own.

The following account is of a personal experience I had in Argentina.

The year was 1980, and the government was a military dictatorship. There was only one gay bar–a dive–in Buenos Aires, a city of 7 million people. The police raided the place so frequently that most gays never went to it. In the absence of a "legal" meeting place, gay men sought one another in public locations, mainly along one of the elegant shopping avenues of the city. Whereas straight men usually avoided the stare of other men, gay men stared back, which was the code used to indicate their interest in each other. One early morning, when I was waiting for a bus, a man walked by and stared at me with intense interest. I stared back. His short hair cut should have alerted me that he was a policeman in civilian clothes out to entrap gays, but before I had time to react he had crossed the street, had approached two policemen in uniform, and had sent them my way. They asked me for my ID. After inspecting it, they told me that I had to go to the police station "por averiguación de antecedentes," to check my police file (everybody in Argentina has a file, even in the absence of criminal activity). At the precinct, they finger printed me, took away my belt and shoe laces so that I could not hang myself, and locked me in a pen with a few drunks and rough guys.

My lover, at the time, expected to meet me that morning in my apartment. When he did not find me there, he called the major hospitals of the area to find out if I had an accident. When he failed to find me that way, he called the municipal morgue, not a crazy idea in a country where people disappeared over night (remember that the phrase "los desaparecidos" originated in Argentina). Finally, he called several police precincts until one of them reported that no information was available, thus confirming I was there. He mobilized his contacts and was able to get me out in a short while. During the hours I spent in the pen, I made up my mind that I would leave Argentina. I did, a year later.

In 1989, I went back. The government was a democracy then. There were gay bars and discos, and Buenos Aires seemed to have caught up with the rest of the civilized world. I saw my former lover again, who offered to show me the new places in town. We went to a couple bars and around 4:00 a.m. ended up in a disco. Ten minutes had scarcely gone by when a few men in civilian clothes demanded that we follow them to the bathroom. There, they showed police badges and asked to see our documents. After almost a decade of life in the U.S., I had grown unaccustomed to carrying documents with me at all times, and I did not have them. Once again, I was arrested.

Years of living in the U.S. plus my U.S. citizenship had made me less docile. I asked to speak with the U.S. ambassador, but they denied me permission. I refused to be put in a pen or be fingerprinted. They made me wait for several hours until finally, at 9:00 a.m., I was taken to see the main officer. He was surrounded by the people in charge of the raid the night before. He screamed at me that I was interfering with the process of justice not allowing them to fingerprint me, and that until that was done he would not listen to me. I was taken back to the detention area and, this time, I allowed them to fingerprint me. While this was being done, one officer casually discussed with a peer how much more he preferred blow jobs from transvestites than from women.

Five hours later, the report from the central Police Department arrived confirming that I had no criminal record. I was taken again to see the main officer. This time, he was alone and calmer than before. He asked me to sit down, and explained to me that this procedure was a routine, that either their division, which I was then informed was the Narcotics Division, or the Morality Division, often raided bars, particularly those frequented by homosexuals. He added, sarcastically, that he had no way of knowing if I was one of them. He asked me what my occupation was. I said I conducted AIDS research with homosexual men in the U.S. He said that that was my problem, that I had lived in the U.S. for too long. I left the country two days later, promising that only under extreme circumstances would I return.

In some cases, police persecution was invoked by homosexuals as a reason to seek asylum in the U.S. One successful case of this type occurred in 1994. In making his case, the man testified:

As I was growing up in Coahuila, Mexico, the police arrested me for walking in certain neighborhoods, patronizing certain bars, and attending certain parties. They falsely accused me of crimes and extorted money from me. . . . When I was a teenager, a friend and I were stopped by police officers. They told my friend to go home and get some money if he wanted to see me again. While my friend was gone, one officer raped me. ("Gay man," 1994)

Later in the article, the gay man's lawyer reports that the U.S. immigration service had been given evidence of the involvement of the police and military authorities in the slaying of homosexuals and doctors working against AIDS in certain parts of Mexico.

Similarly, a *Chicago Tribune* article (Marx, 1992) quoted a gay activist who denounced that 40 male prostitutes, transvestites, and gays had been murdered in the prior two years by right-wing groups and leftist Tupac Amaru Revolutionary Movement guerrillas seeking to "clean up the streets." The same article reports the claim of gay activists that paramilitary squads linked to police and narcotraffickers killed at least 320 male prostitutes, transvestites, and gays in Colombia over a seven year period, and similar groups in Brazil killed more than 710 male prostitutes, transvestites, and gays since 1980, according to Brazilian newspaper reports.

Canada is another country that granted asylum to a homosexual fleeing persecution in his country, this time Argentina ("Gay argentino gana su caso . . . , " *Opinión Cultural,* 1-92).

It is clear that not every homosexual in Latin America has been a direct victim of police harassment. Yet, the examples presented, reports we heard from different countries, and those told by other authors (Lumsden, 1991) are strikingly similar. Those individuals who have not themselves been prey of the police know about the abuses and live their lives with the fear of being the next victim.

The widespread feeling in the population is that there is nowhere to appeal to right a wrong: the government is perceived as corrupt from the top down, and this perception may not be inaccurate. Let us just remember that in the 90s, Mexico's former president (Salinas) was accused of links to those who killed an opponent presidential candidate, the president of Colombia (Samper) was shown to have received funds from drug traffickers for his election campaign, a former president of Brazil (Collor) had to resign under corruption charges, and the former head of the armed forces and former president of Chile (Pinochet) has kept a prominent government role despite clear links to assassin movements that wiped out the opposition. This does not even take into account the many decades of corrupt military governments that preceded the current administrations.

HOMOPHOBIA IN MENTAL HEALTH

Latin American psychology and psychotherapy are strongly influenced by European schools, particularly psychoanalysis. Although in recent decades U.S. schools of psychology have become better known, the change is taking place slowly. From a psychoanalytic perspective, homosexuality is understood as a fixation in the psychosexual development of a person and, consequently, a pathology. Many practitioners continue to hold to this view, most likely in consonance with their own prejudices. I remember a session that took place in my early twenties when, full of anxiety, I discussed with my psychotherapist someone's comment that it was a waste of time for me to try to be a psychotherapist when I was going to be unable to help a patient move beyond the developmental point in which I was fixated. My therapist replied, "That is not completely true," which of course left room for me to think that there was some truth to the statement and that I was doomed to professional failure.

When they come out, many men, particularly young ones, are taken by relatives to see a psychotherapist. The likelihood of the therapist being gay-affirmative is quite small, and this may result in a negative experience that may taint future attempts at psychotherapy as well. A Dominican man who participated in one of my studies told me, with great distress, his experience undergoing aversive therapy at the Clínica de Psicología de la Universidad Autónoma de Santo Domingo. During the therapeutic sessions, he was encouraged to get aroused looking at pictures of nude males. Subsequently, he was administered electric discharges in the pelvis so as to create a negative association. The patient was 17 years old when fifteen sessions of this treatment took place. He was told that a vomitive substance could be used instead of electricity if the latter did not work. The patient was encouraged to get married to a woman, which he did. The marriage lasted less than three years. Looking back at his experience, this man, currently an open homosexual, states that he underwent "psychiatric torture."

INSUFFICIENT ORGANIZATION
OF THE GAY COMMUNITY

Homosexual activity in the Americas can be traced to the time of the Aztecs (Kimball, 1993). Attempts to organize homosexual groups appeared in the 1970s in Argentina (Anabiarte & Lorenzo, 1979) and in Mexico (Lumsden, 1991). These attempts were generally linked to leftist movements who advocated freedom for oppressed minorities. They generally encountered strong governmental opposition, especially in countries with right-wing dictatorships like Argentina. Although the political climate changed in the 1980s and many countries reverted to democracies, the general attitude against homosexual organizations still prevails.

A telling case is the three-year struggle for legal recognition suffered by the Comunidad Homosexual Argentina. The request had initially been backed by human rights organizations and the Department of Civil Associations of the Justice Department. Yet, that same department later rejected the request stating that it could not make place for "a hybrid third gender." When this decision was appealed, the judges stated that legal recognition was denied to the association based on "its stated purpose of public defense of homosexuality." When the president of Argentina, Carlos Menem, was confronted by homosexual activists during a presentation at Columbia University in New York, he instructed his collaborators to intercede in favor of the homosexual organization. The Argentine Supreme Court denied legal status to the organization stating, "the Christian morality rejects this type of behavior that goes against the purpose of reproduction of the species." After further struggles, the Association was finally legally recognized on March 19, 1992 ("Obtuvo su personería jurídica," 1992).

In other countries, one could find *un ambiente gay* (a gay milieu) rather than an organized gay community. Reporting on gay life in Brazil, Parker (1991) writes,

> It is only in the very recent past that anything remotely similar to a "gay community" can be found in the most modern areas of some Brazilian cities, and even here, the notion that homosexuality might serve as the focus for a political movement is clearly limited to a very small segment of the elite.

In Mexico, some organizations such as the Grupo Orgullo Homosexual Liberación, in Guadalajara, achieved some leverage in their dealings with police and civic authorities, but changing political climates took a serious toll on the progress made (Carrier, 1995; Wilson, 1995). Gay organizations seem to be limited to Mexico City and Guadalajara (Lumsden, 1991).

It appears safe to state that gay life in most Latin American countries is in transition from a stage of informal organizations focused mainly on entertainment to one of political activism in which the defense of the groups' civil rights and the progress of the community are the primary goals. Gay organizations in most Latin American countries are not in the latter stage yet, and their activities generally take place only in the most important urban centers. As a result, individuals who experience same sex attraction still face isolation and little support and validation of their feelings from peers who are "out and proud."

TRANSGRESSION AS A SURVIVAL MECHANISM

We see, therefore, that Latin American homosexuals must confront a society with strong gender stereotypes, a homophobic Catholic church that actively campaigns against homosexuals, actual or feared extortion in the hands of the police, and mental health professionals who continue to define homosexuality as a pathology, all the while lacking the support of organized gay agencies that could act in their defense. Faced with these accumulated negative pressures on one side, and with undeniable homosexual tendencies on the other, homosexual men in Latin America developed survival strategies based mainly on transgression. Transgression is doing what one was told not to do. Where a rule was laid down forbidding men from living their sexuality openly, homosexuals found ways to circumvent the prohibition. The popular child's game *policía y ladrón* (police and thieves), became reenacted as an adult game in which homosexuals took chances trying to achieve the desired goals regardless of prohibitions. Transgression, of course, is not limited to homosexuals: It is another manifestation of the habitual survival strategies employed by men and women of Latin American societies to deal with the corrupt systems in power.

Among homosexuals, transgressions range from the maintenance of another man's gaze to signal a personal interest, to overt defiance of prohibitions by gathering in known cruising areas or holding gay parties while bribing the infiltrated police. Transgression is present at a more intimate sexual level, as violation of cultural taboos with its ensuing pleasure. Parker (1996) writes,

> Throughout Latin America, a strong emphasis is placed on the transgression of socially sanctioned norms as a key element in the very definition of erotically satisfying sexual relations, and a range of sexual practices associated with increased risk for HIV transmission (such as both heterosexual and homosexual

anal intercourse) play a special role in the definition of sexual or erotic scripts. (p. 63)

MIGRATION

Migration to "the North" is another strategy employed by those homosexuals who find intolerable the repression in their countries of origin. These homosexuals often chose San Francisco or New York City as a destination given the purported tolerant attitudes of those cities.

Migration is not an easy step. It takes plenty of courage to leave behind family, friends, and familiar surroundings to establish oneself in a different environment, with a new language and unfamiliar rules of functioning. It also takes money, and for many immigrants this means selling all their possessions or gathering funds from family members that will painstakingly be returned at a later date. Except for Puerto Ricans, all other Latin Americans face immigration hurdles before entering the U.S. Participants in our studies have related months of traveling through different Latin American countries trying to reach Mexico, and then anxiously waiting near the frontier until, in the middle of the night, with the help of a *coyote,* they could enter the U.S. Others came with student visas that they let expire, with fake work contracts, with requests from fake relatives, etc. In other words, transgression was, once again, the means to achieve the goal.

After this protracted effort, when the immigrant homosexual men reach the gay meccas of the North, they feel fascinated by the possibilities: Spread-out gay neighborhoods, sex shops with windows on the sidewalk selling erotic paraphernalia, free weekly magazines displaying publicity for sex clubs illustrated with semi-nude men, theaters that advertise on their marquees all male shows, peep rooms with back rooms, plus a wide variety of public meeting places where men cruise openly. It is not difficult to realize that in such enticing environment, far from the repressive elements operating back home, men may wish to indulge in a feast of sexual experiences. There is one caveat, though: The rampant AIDS epidemic requires that sex follow certain rules known as safer-sex. At this point, the old behavioral patterns come into play again. Men who grew up hearing that they should not have certain types of sex (with other men) are told once again that certain sexual acts are to be avoided ("Avoid anal sex," "Use a condom every time"). Although the circumstances have changed and the men can appreciate the difference between a repressive society and a viral epidemic, the experience is the same: sexual expression has to be curtailed and done according to someone else's guidelines. The medical authority steps into the role previously occupied by the church and the police. And once again the strategy to deal with it is transgression paired with the hope of not getting infected with HIV.

The situation described above should help explain why certain prevention strategies and psychotherapeutic modalities that are fruitful when applied to European American gay men, do not necessarily work well with Latin American MSM. The latter have been subject to many traumatic experiences that have resulted in behavioral patterns to deal with oppression, harassment, and discrimination and that now interfere with a rational, straightforward adherence to prevention messages.

Although migration to the U.S. opens plenty of new possibilities, many Latin American men cannot free themselves from the oppressive past. Often, they continue to live in neighborhoods populated by co-nationals who hold the same prejudices they had in their native countries. For example, a Dominican man who participated in one of my studies reported that he went to see a Latino physician in New York City to consult him about erection difficulties he was experiencing as a result of the blood pressure medication he was taking. The physician, knowing that his patient was homosexual, asked him why he was bothered about not having an erection since he did not need it (implying that homosexuals only get penetrated). In other cases, Latin American men continue to feel paranoid about possible disclosures to family members, even if they live in a different country: their feeling is that there could always be someone who knows someone else who knows their family. Furthermore, in the face of racism and discrimination towards minorities in the U.S. these men continue to be guarded and distrustful of the social environment. Only a selected few are able to integrate themselves into mainstream communities, especially the organized European American gay community. This integration is generally contingent on having white skin, being well educated, and being able to use English almost as well as a native. These same prerequisites for integration apply to men of Latin American descent born in the U.S.

DISCUSSION AND SUGGESTIONS FOR PREVENTION

Current HIV prevention trends in the European American gay community consist of refining the target of intervention and developing population-specific programs. One such strategy is to focus on HIV-negative gay men. These men have felt almost forgotten in a milieu where most of the attention was paid to peers who were infected or dying. Many of these HIV-negative men felt almost embarrassed about voicing their needs, and some even thought that seroconversion was a way of belonging to the community. Given this situation, programs centered on HIV-negative men make a lot of sense.

Except for fully integrated and assimilated Latin American men, this scenario is probably not pertinent to this group. One cannot feel left out if one was never in. And before Latin American men can feel part of a gay community, they need to deal with the sequelae of their oppressive past and the social realities of their present environment.

Dealing with the past will be an arduous process. It will require becoming aware of internalized homophobic feelings and how they impact on present behaviors. At an individual level, these men may be aided by psychotherapeutic work with therapists aware of the pressures that affected their clients' lives while growing up in Latin America. The work of the therapist will not be easy. Often, internalized homophobia is so deeply ingrained in the individual that he is not aware of it. It may also have been sublimated into personal characteristics that the individual considers virtues. For example, a long time psychotherapeutic patient of mine kept postponing the fulfillment of his needs, to the point of not even having a room of his own, while his brothers, with whom he worked in a family owned property, progressively secured for themselves and their families spacious apartments. My patient kept justifying his situation, claiming that, since he was not married and had no children, he wanted to allow his siblings to take care of their needs. Yet, under this supposedly generous behavior, there lurked the feeling that, being homosexual, he did not deserve anything.

Besides psychotherapy, involvement with other gay men, discussion of past experiences, and mutual support may help Latino men to critically analyze their past and shed negative associations. This may also be a source of strength to deal with the stressors they experience in their present lives, such as economic inequalities, racism, and discrimination. But there is the danger that peer involvement will be reduced to group socializing without promoting community development. In this respect, the theories of the Brazilian educator Paulo Freire and his recommendations concerning critical consciousness development (*concientización*) may be very helpful (Freire, 1990). He postulated that all human beings, no matter how oppressed they may be, are capable of looking critically at their world in a dialectic encounter with others. Provided with the proper analytic tools to question his or her circumstances, an individual can gradually perceive his or her personal and social reality as well as the contradictions in it, become conscious of his or her own perception of that reality, and deal critically with it. Freire postulates that the old, paternalistic teacher-student or top-down relationship must be overcome and replaced by a process in which education takes place between peers. In this process of liberation, "those who have been completely marginalized are so radically transformed [that] they are no longer willing to be mere objects, responding to changes occurring around them; they are more likely to decide to take upon themselves the struggle to change the structures of society which until now have served to oppress them" (p. 14).

A number of Latino gay organizations have appeared in the U.S. in the last decade, generally in relation to AIDS prevention. There is one national level organization, the National Latino Lesbian and Gay Organization (LLEGO), which promotes local initiatives. These organizations have the potential (and the immense challenge) of counteracting the influence of the negative factors described above by presenting positive Latino gay role models, encouraging gay pride, and offering forums to question the homophobic mores in which Latino men were raised. If, within their culture, Latino gay men were made to feel weak, sinful, criminal, and ill, the time has come for them to shed these prejudices, not because someone else tells them to do so, but because in analyzing such concepts they are found wanting. Once this process has taken place, Latino MSM will be free from internal oppression so as to question their past and present societies and their repressive mechanisms. These men will then have the tools to demand respect and equality, not only at an individual level but also as a group. And they will be able to protect themselves and their partners from HIV-infection, because they will feel collectively entitled to life.

REFERENCES

Anabiarte, H., & Lorenzo, R. (1979). Homosexualidad: El asunto está caliente. In H. Anabiarte & R. Lorenzo (Eds.), *Persecución y muerte en el mundo cristiano*. Madrid. Queimada Ediciones.

Arenas, R., & Koch, D. M. (1994). *Before night falls*. New York: Penguin USA.

Cáceres, C., & Rosasco, A. M. (1993). An HIV/STD prevention program for homosexually active men of diverse sexual identities. Presented at the IX International Conference on AIDS in Berlin.

Canada: Gay argentino gana su caso de refugio. (Canada: Gay Argentine wins refugee case). (1992, January). *Opinión Cultural, 4*(1), p. 32.

Carballo-Diéguez, A. (1992). *Towards an emic typology of Latino men who have sex with men. Abstracts of the VII International Conference of AIDS/III STD World Congress*. Amsterdam, The Netherlands, POD-5176.

Carballo-Diéguez, A., & Dolezal, C. (1995). Association between history of childhood sexual abuse and adult HIV-risk sexual behavior in Puerto Rican men who have sex with men. *Child Abuse & Neglect, The International Journal, 19*(5), 595-605.

Carrier, J. M. (1977). "Sex-role preference" as an explanatory variable in homosexual behavior. *Archives of Sexual Behavior, 6*(1), 53-65.

Carrier, J. (1995). *De los otros: Intimacy and homosexuality among Mexican men*. New York: Columbia University Press.

Culturelinc Corporation. (1991). *Cultural factors among Hispanics: Perception and prevention of HIV infection*. Available from NYSDOH, phone # (516) 473-0139.

de la Cancela, V. (1986). A critical analysis of Puerto Rican machismo: Implications for clinical practice. *Psychotherapy, 23*(2), 291-296.

de la Cancela, V. (1989). Minority AIDS prevention: Moving beyond cultural perspectives towards sociopolitical empowerment. *AIDS Education and Prevention, 1*(2), 141-153.

Escobar, G. (1994, September 24). Cardinal's comment on gays backfires in Argentina. *The Washington Post*, p. A23.

Freire, P. (1990). *Pedagogy of the oppressed*. New York, NY: Continuum Publishing Company.

Fry, P. (1984-85). Male homosexuality and spirit possession in Brazil. *Journal of Homosexuality, 10-11*, 137-153.

Gay Man Who Cited Abuse in Mexico Is Granted Asylum. (1994, March 26). *New York Times*, p. 6.

Guillén, L. (1994). Gladys. In L. Guillén (Ed.), *Soy homosexual.* (pp. 21-25). Mexico, DF: Del Milenio.

Kimball, G. (1993). Aztec homosexuality: The textual evidence. *Journal of Homosexuality, 26*(1), 7-24.

Lancaster, R. N. (1988). Subject honor and object shame: The construction of male homosexuality and stigma in Nicaragua. *Ethnology, 27*(2), 111-125.

Lumsden, I. (1991). *Homosexuality: Society and the state in Mexico.* Toronto: Canadian Gay Archives.

Marx, G. (1992, January 28). Gays in Latin America begin to claim rights. *Chicago Tribune*, p. 1.

Mexican archbishop lashes out at homosexuals. (1991). *Reuters.* Mexico City.

Muñoz, E. (1996). The little devil. In R. González (Ed.), *Muy macho: Latino men confront their manhood.* New York: Doubleday.

New York City Department of Health, Bureau of Disease Intervention Research. (May 1995). Men who have sex with men (MSM). Work Group, prepared for PPG95.

Obtuvo su personería jurídica la Comunidad Homosexual Argentino Una batalla legal de tres años. (The Argentine homosexual community obtained its legal recognition. A three year battle). (1992, March). *Clarin.*

Parker, R. (1986). Masculinity, femininity, and homosexuality: On the anthropological interpretation of sexual meanings in Brazil. *Journal of Homosexuality, 11*, 155-163.

Parker, R. G. (1996). Behaviour in Latin American men: Implications for HIV/ AIDS interventions. *International Journal of STD & AIDS, 7*(2), 62-65.

Parker, R. G. (1991). *Bodies, pleasures, and passions: Sexual culture in contemporary Brazil.* Boston, MA: Beacon Press.

Paz, O. (1993). *El laberinto de la soledad, postdata y vuelta a el laberinto de la soledad* (pp. 33-71). Mexico, DF: Fondo de Cultura Economica, S.A. De C.V. Mascaras Mexicanas.

Ramírez, R. (1993). *Dime Capitán: Reflexiones sobre la masculinidad.* Río Piedras, P.R.: Ediciones Huracán.

Sandoval, L. V. (June, 1995). Homosexuales al altar. *Rumbo*, 9-15.

Schifter-Sikora, J. (1989). *Homosexualismo y SIDA en Costa Rica.* Quayacán, S.A.

Wilson, C. (1995). *Hidden in the blood: A personal investigation of AIDS in the Yucatán.* New York: Columbia University Press.

CONCEPTS AND THE FUTURE

Discursive Condoms in the Age of AIDS: Queer(y)ing HIV Prevention

Peter A. Newman

SUMMARY. This article applies queer theory in a critical approach to AIDS. While extant psychosocial literature on HIV/AIDS focuses almost exclusively on the biomedical epidemic of disease, AIDS discourse is also a crucial arena for investigation. The concepts of minoritizing, universalizing, and heteronormativity that inform a queer theoretical perspective will first be explicated in application to sexual orientation. These concepts will then be deployed in elucidating a series of intersections and confounds among sexuality, identity, and

Peter A. Newman is a doctoral candidate in the combined program of social work and psychology at the University of Michigan.

The author expresses his gratitude to Anne Herrmann, Beth Glover Reed, Pat Simons and Larry Gant of the University of Michigan, and to Michael Shernoff, for stimulation, dialogue and support. Special thanks also goes to Steve Ball for providing detailed feedback and editorial suggestions.

In memory of Stephen Carter, 1964-1994.

[Haworth co-indexing entry note]: "Discursive Condoms in the Age of AIDS: Queer(y)ing HIV Prevention." Newman, Peter A. Co-published simultaneously in *Journal of Gay & Lesbian Social Services* (The Haworth Press, Inc.) Vol. 8, No. 1, 1998, pp. 83-102; and: *The HIV-Negative Gay Man: Developing Strategies for Survival and Emotional Well-Being* (ed: Steven Ball) The Haworth Press, Inc., 1998, pp. 83-102; and: *The HIV-Negative Gay Man: Developing Strategies for Survival and Emotional Well-Being* (ed: Steven Ball) The Harrington Park Press, an imprint of The Haworth Press, Inc., 1998, pp. 83-102. Single or multiple copies of this article are available for a fee from The Haworth Document Delivery Service [1-800-342-9678, 9:00 a.m. - 5:00 p.m. (EST). E-mail address: getinfo@haworth.com].

83

HIV/AIDS, that result in tremendous problems for prevention. Ostensible prevention messages will be shown at times, paradoxically, to encourage HIV promotion. Critical analysis and investigation of AIDS and HIV prevention discourse are advocated as a proactive strategy for helping HIV-negative gay men and gay male youth to remain HIV-negative. *[Article copies available for a fee from The Haworth Document Delivery Service: 1-800-342-9678. E-mail address: getinfo@haworth.com]*

The gay and lesbian community has been a pioneer in HIV prevention efforts and the inventor of safer sex. The complexities and paradoxes of AIDS, and its prevention, however, continue to confound and elude even our most well-intentioned endeavors. As rates of new seroconversions for HIV are leveling off (still amounting to tens of thousands of new cases each year) or declining for some of the population–injection drug users, and adult gay men–they continue to escalate among people of color, youth, and particularly among gay youth and gay youth of color (Fleming, 1996; Odets, 1994). It is estimated that one in four new cases of HIV infection is among youth aged 13 to 20 years old (Fleming, 1996). The mean life expectancy for a gay male youth in San Francisco (one of the few locales where data on gay youth are collected) aged 16 to 24, is 45 years old (Odets, 1994).

A substantial proportion of new seroconversions among gay men is in the younger generation. But we have no cause for complacency in addressing adult gay men either. What was once thought to be inexorable and indelible progress in the implementation of safer sex by adult gay men has been called into question with an apparent return to unsafe sexual practices by formerly "safe" men–what has been called "relapse" or "recidivism" (Stall et al., 1990). This terminology has appropriately been challenged as it tacitly pathologizes and criminalizes sex between men (Hart & Boulton, 1995).

Given the continuing new seroconversions among gay men, it is clear that those of us committed to the health and well-being of this population must approach prevention anew. The context in which prevention strategies were formulated in 1984 is no longer operative in 1998. For one, it has become increasingly evident that HIV is not a temporary phenomenon. Initially, safer sex was not conceptualized with a lifetime in mind (Shernoff, personal communication).

Yet a decade and a half into the pandemic, the magic bullet continues to elude us; it appears likely that safer sex will remain an institution. A second major change impacting prevention is that there is now a widely available and much touted test for the HIV antibody that, for those who are tested, enables us to discern who has the HIV antibody and who does not (Odets, 1994). Together these shifts speak to a vastly different context for understanding HIV and its prevention.

Our current knowledge about HIV related risk taking behavior has been informed by a plethora of correlational studies of psychosocial risks for serotransmission undertaken in the last decade. While such studies may have initially augmented our knowledge, they offer little in the way of exploring the mechanisms and meanings underlying the linkages they describe (*why* do younger gay men engage in more unprotected anal sex than older gay men?; *why* do they use condoms less consistently?), or in progressing to strategies for preventive intervention. In fact, correlational studies often feed misconceptions which result in the naturalizing of AIDS as a disease of the 'gay male body,' and as somehow inherent according to a variety of other social categorizations as well–along the lines of race, age, and gender.

The main contention of this article is that we must critically approach AIDS, and HIV prevention, to address the problem of the continued serotransmission of HIV among gay men. It is essential that we unpack the various meanings which have been inscribed on HIV/AIDS. I will argue that in the apprehensive aftermath of the sexual revolution of the late 1960s and early 1970s, in the post-Stonewall era in which homosexuality *per se* was finally deleted as a pathology in the *Diagnostic and Statistical Manual of Mental Disorders,* AIDS functioned as a fantasized marker for gay men.

The test for HIV–tellingly misunderstood as 'the AIDS test'–offered a fantasized and scientifically mythologized method for identifying and re-pathologizing the homosexual other. Reframing HIV/AIDS from this perspective enables us to explore present conundrums regarding the continued seroconversions of gay men in a new light. To this end, I will employ a perspective which is derived from queer theory.

Queer theory, in both its newness and its radical positioning, is not (and cannot be) a pre-ordained and agreed upon "school of thought." There are concepts, however, that are characteristic of this mode of inquiry. I will begin by explicating the terms minoritizing, universalizing, and heteronormativity. Next I will apply these concepts to an investigation of the history and discourse (the language, texts, and meanings) of AIDS. I will then use a queer theoretical perspective to elicit some of the intransigent problems and paradoxes in the messages of HIV prevention–messages which may appear at first to be unidimensional and unproblematic. The question driving this investigation is how we might re-approach and recalibrate HIV prevention for gay men and gay male youth in light of insights gleaned from a critical re-thinking of AIDS.

MINORITIZING/UNIVERSALIZING/HETERONORMATIVITY

Minoritizing and universalizing, key concepts in queer theory, can be most clearly explained by way of application. Sexual orientation, for example, can be understood from both perspectives. From a minoritizing point of view, gay men, lesbians, and bisexuals compose a unique minority in the American population–sometimes seen as having occupied this position across time, and across cultures. As a distinct subpopulation, nonheterosexuals represent a different group from that of the dominant heterosexual culture.

From a universalizing perspective, we are all "polymorphously perverse." Each individual has the potential for homosexual, bisexual, and heterosexual outcomes–to apply our currently naturalized taxonomy. As we each have in us seeds for a variety of sexual orientations, and even may foreclose on attaining any fixed outcome, it becomes misleading to speak of a minority. What seems unique and deviant is really universal.

Another important concept in a queer theoretical perspective, and one that is directly related to the minoritizing/universalizing discussion, is heteronormativity. Heteronormativity is somewhat distinct from homophobia and heterosexism, and takes us further in the exploration of anti-gay attitudes and acts. While homophobia suggests the irrational fear and hatred of gay men and lesbians (Weinberg, 1973), and heterosexism is directed more at the institutionalization of anti-gay attitudes in social programs, policies, and law

(Neisen, 1990), heteronormativity defines the entire context in which gay/lesbian/bisexual is seen as marked and marginal (Sedgwick, 1990). From a heteronormative perspective, and even absent manifest and recognizable homophobia and heterosexism, nonheterosexuality is always conceptualized as aberrant. Even the most well-meaning theorist or researcher who may "sympathize" with the "plight" of gay men and lesbians, may nonetheless operate with the unquestioned understanding that upholds heterosexuality as more natural, viable, and normal than nonheterosexuality. Emblematic of heteronormativity is an obsessive search for the cause(s) of homosexuality. Interestingly, heteronormativity can be seen to operate whether this search is situated in either the nature or the nurture camp. "It's due to socialization," or "it's in the genes" both nonetheless seek to explain a phenomenon seen as abnormal and thus requiring an etiological explanation.

Heteronormativity calls attention to the power relationship between heterosexuality and queerness, that valorizes and naturalizes heterosexuality. In fact, 'homosexuality' preceded 'heterosexuality' in defining identities based on sexual object choice (Foucault, 1978). Homosexuality becomes necessary in supporting the fiction of a normal, universal, and natural heterosexuality. In adopting a perspective that challenges heteronormativity, one may then be at least equally pressed in investigating what causes heterosexuality; or, perhaps more vitally, what causes homophobia and heterosexism.

The concepts of minoritizing and universalizing, as well as heteronormativity, offer different ways of conceptualizing sexual orientation. What is crucial–and I will extend this to HIV prevention–is that apparently similar terms and messages can have dramatically different meanings depending on the perspective through which one understands HIV/AIDS and sexuality. The minoritizing/ universalizing dichotomy also enables us to evaluate our comprehension of the relationship between identity and behavior, which is central to how we understand and approach AIDS.

IDENTITY/BEHAVIOR

A minoritizing view tends to extol identity. Identity is seen as explaining, in and of itself, a variety of thoughts, feelings, behaviors, and fantasies. From a universalizing position, we can ask how it is that certain behaviors or features–and not others–become consolidated in what becomes a coherent identity. Why is it that sexual orientation is defined around one's sexual object choice, rather than one's desires for different sexual acts, for example? Or, why have sexual orientation, or skin color, become such potent criteria for social identity categorization, as opposed to height, food preferences, or eye color?

In regard to sexuality, Foucault (1978) argued that while sodomy had existed for centuries, only in the late 19th century with the ascendancy of the field of sexology–a new 'science' of sex–did a whole new (heretofore undifferentiated) species of persons become identified in the sodomite. Foucault discusses the shift from conceiving of sexuality as a compendium of acts to conceptualizing a field of sexual types embodied in distinct persons. This change enabled a project of control over the realm of (what was now understood to be) sexuality. Individual persons could be situated and cited as deviant. Previously there existed the idea that all individuals were more or less capable of engaging in what may have been understood as perverse sexual acts. This paradigm shift, and the tensions that persevere in the differing understandings of sexuality that ensue, can be seen to operate powerfully in our understandings and confusions around HIV/AIDS. "To be gay, or to be potentially classifiable as gay . . . in this system is to come under the radically overlapping aegises of a universalizing discourse of acts or bonds and a minoritizing discourse of kinds of persons" (Sedgwick, 1990, p. 54).

Questioning the fixity of the meaning of concepts such as sexual orientation, heterosexual, gay, and lesbian, allows us to critically approach AIDS. The identity categories, in a minoritizing view, that become connected to HIV/AIDS are neither spontaneous nor random; neither, of course, are they necessarily aligned with AIDS. Minoritizing and universalizing perspectives can help us to revisit what is often taken for granted in AIDS-sexuality-identity-behavior connections, and to pose questions such as the following: How has AIDS become coterminous with the gay male body, and also signified along racial and ethnic lines? What are the dynamics which motivate a minoritizing perspective of identities in application to

AIDS–as opposed to a universalizing focus on behaviors–and which serve to construct AIDS as a disease of particular kinds of people? These are crucial questions for an interrogation of prevention.

From a universalizing vantage point, HIV is an equal opportunity infectious agent. A virus knows no morals. When bodily and environmental conditions are right, transmission may occur. Of course this includes the fact that at least one partner must be HIV-positive. From a universalizing stance there exists a ubiquitous potentiality for HIV transmission that is wholly non-contingent on identity. Identity categorizations, for example risk group status, are challenged as naïve and rather transparent means of approaching safer sex. And even more than forcing the issue that transmission is a function of behavior–anyone's behavior–a universalizing position highlights viral transmission as a stochastic process. It is impossible to accurately predict during which specific encounters viral transmission will in fact occur. Such is the foundation of a universalizing discourse of HIV disease.

A minoritizing view can be seen to arise in part as an attempt to negotiate anxiety. "It is in the world of representations," writes Gilman (1988, p. 107), "that we manage our fear of disease. . . . " Placing blame for catastrophic disease is a way of attempting to defend and immunize oneself against fear. Particularly when a deadly disease remains an enigma to science, when medicine is perceived as impotent, as was characteristic in the early to mid-1980s of what we now know as AIDS, ascribing blame becomes a central strategy for establishing the boundaries of health and illness, the borders of safety and danger. "By drawing firm boundaries–by placing blame on 'other groups' or on 'deviant behavior'–we try to avoid the randomness of disease and dying, to escape from our inherent sense of vulnerability, to exorcise the mortality inherent in the human condition" (Nelkin & Gilman, 1988, p. 378).

Along these lines, it is not surprising, nor is it unique, that in response to AIDS–an initially cryptic disease with the apparent power to kill–categories were constructed to attenuate the fear and anxiety that result. Simple identity-based understandings allow one to compartmentalize danger so as to manage fear. What is striking in the case of AIDS is that once a virus was discovered as the underlying cause of this heretofore unknown disease entity, once science had constructed the basis for a biomedical explanation, sociological explanations persevered as central to the conceptualization of disease. AIDS became hot-wired, so to speak, to the gay male body. It becomes crucial to prevention to explore how gay identity became coterminous with AIDS in the United States. Minoritizing and universalizing perspectives are powerful tools in this endeavor.

From a minoritizing position, the construction of a homosexual other reifies and supports the fiction of a 'normal,' sealed-off heterosexuality. The gay/straight dichotomy also serves to establish the social bounds of appropriate (heterosexual) behavior: It becomes acceptable for a man to touch another man (a behavior potentially indicating that one is gay), for example, if he is protected by a heterosexual identity. The protection offered by a homo/hetero dichotomy is a dual-edged sword, however. There exists a defense against being discredited so long as one is understood to be heterosexual, but there is also an ever-present threat: One is always potentially discreditable (Goffman, 1963) in being indicted (perhaps in both legal and more figurative uses of the word) as queer. To the extent to which one can't tell who is gay and who is straight, the specter of universalism remains haunting. The history, in U.S. military policy, of obsessive interpellation of gays and lesbians (when not in wartime), and the now ludicrous "Don't Ask, Don't Tell," are emblematic of this fear.

Understood in the context of the tremendous tensions extant in the gay/straight dichotomy, AIDS offered apparently visible signs of one's being gay and, more importantly, signs whose intelligibility was undergirded by the *sine qua non* of a scientific lexicon. HIV was deployed in an attempt to realign the unstable hierarchy as to the moral rectitude and the ascendancy of heterosexuality. Beyond the insistent iterations of sociological explanations for a viral entity—perfectly captured in the longevity in the media and the dominant heterosexual imagery of "GRID" (gay-related immune deficiency) and "gay plague," to say nothing of "WOGS" (the wrath of God syndrome)—the obsession with, and the overwhelming resources poured into HIV testing provide further evidence for the perceived threat to heteronormativity that queers represented. A focus on discerning who is HIV-positive and who is HIV-negative, as opposed to one on implementing behavioral risk reduction, is emblematic of a minoritizing discourse of identities in the AIDS arena.

The 'AIDS test,' then, offered a powerful discursive condom–an imagined protection (in language and thought) against both AIDS and homosexuality. It is within this larger discursive context that HIV disease, and, perhaps more critically, HIV prevention, must be re-assessed.

HIV-POSITIVE/HIV-NEGATIVE

One powerful effect of the HIV antibody test is that a new class of identity is engendered in HIV-positive and HIV-negative. Persons with no other ostensible differences (or similarities) than the results of an ELISA test–persons who may be equally (or unequally) healthy/unhealthy, strong/weak, young/old and, paradoxically, gay/straight, black/white, male/female–come to share a new identity constituted by the detection/non-detection of a viral antibody. In this schema, HIV-negative gay men come to be defined by an absence, even as this is an absence of a potentially deadly virus. Given the media attention and community support focused, until the recent present (see Johnston, 1995; Odets, 1995), almost exclusively on the plight of HIV-positive gay men, feeling oneself an outsider is not an unusual experience among HIV-negative gay men. This feeling is ever more potent as it rekindles the alienation experienced by perhaps many gay men in their youth. Feeling alienated from the larger heterosexual population by virtue of being queer is reproduced, and precisely in that which previously had been a haven of security and belonging–in the gay community. A powerful and contentious field of identity politics emerged out of the signification of HIV serostatus. The instantiation of this difference, its power to arouse and enrage, is eloquently captured in several recent texts (Odets, 1995; Rofes, 1996; Sadownick, 1995; Warner, 1995a).

Given the potency of the HIV-positive/HIV-negative dichotomy, and the fiery emotionality it engages, it is imperative that serostatus be addressed in interrogating prevention. In the larger population, the HIV antibody test may have served as a signifier of sexual difference; seropositivity was aligned with being queer. In the gay community, these minoritizing boundaries are simulated and reproduced, and have similarly created divisions and distinct identities. These are seen in distinct support groups for HIV-positive and HIV-negative gay men, dances and social events designed for HIV-positive gay men, and the People with AIDS Coalition, for example. This is not at all to suggest anything wrong with these activities; rather, these examples serve to underscore the power of HIV-negative/HIV-positive in fostering distinct identities.

There also exist powerful echoes of the closet in the fears and feelings that accompany disclosure of one's HIV status–and this exists for positives as well as negatives. Identifying as HIV-positive or HIV-negative may be empowering or alienating, marginalizing or enfranchising–along both sides of the divide; but nowhere does it engender such violent incoherences and deadly confusion as in the messages of HIV prevention. Here identity-based claims based on one's being HIV-positive or HIV-negative serve as an often apocryphal (and deadly wrong) prevention strategy predicated on the ability to be able to 'tell' (who is HIV-positive/HIV-negative).

A new field of understanding is mobilized in identifying persons as HIV-positive or HIV-negative, which in turn fosters a means of approaching safer sex through partner selection. This can be contrasted with a universalizing strategy which would advocate unilateral precautions when engaging in any sexual activity deemed as risky. As we shall see, neither strategy offers a perfect solution; nor is it my goal to adjudicate between the two. Rather, due to competing minoritizing and universalizing views, differing conceptualizations–seen in gay/straight, identity/behavior, and HIV-positive/HIV-negative–the messages, language, and meanings most often deployed in HIV prevention often break down into incoherence and paradox.

QUEER(Y)ING HIV PREVENTION

A variety of problems in meaning and understanding in the domain of HIV prevention can be shown to emerge out of competing universalizing and minoritizing conceptualizations of sexuality. Much of the difficulty in helping HIV-negative men to remain HIV-negative also arises out of the heteronormative assumptions that are structured into our understanding of AIDS and sexuality. Embedded in some of our most well-intentioned prevention efforts are the very seeds for exacerbating the epidemic. To the extent that the gay = AIDS equation has persevered, this identity-based fantasy of prevention lapses into a nightmare of confusion.

I will now explore the differences in meaning that may be derived from apparently unidimensional messages depending on one's frame of understanding. In each case I will present a prevention message, and then problematize it from a variety of perspectives that may evoke the gay/straight, identity/behavior and HIV-negative/HIV-positive binarisms. It is crucial that we develop the ability to read the minoritizing/universalizing tensions in a given text so as to anticipate the confusion and subversion that are sometimes inherent, and to militate against the homophobia and heteronormativity extant in the language of some of our prevention messages. It is from these possibilities of differential understandings and interpretations for which the stage has now been set, that I envision new prevention strategies for gay men and gay male youth in the 1990s.

From a universalizing standpoint, safer sex makes sense. As HIV transmission is a function of behaviors in which there is risk of transfer of blood, semen, and/or vaginal fluid, barrier methods of protection would seem to be indicated. *Use a condom every time.* To the extent, however, that 'gay sex' is risky sex—a conflation of behavior and identity—'heterosexual sex' is safer sex. Sex between gay men becomes necessarily risky. Hence, the loaded and dangerously distorted, *Know your partner.* But to the extent that being a gay man means having (had) sex with other gay men, *being gay* is *a priori* risky. So, use a condom every time—regardless as to whether one's partner is HIV-positive or negative. Alternatively, why use a condom if one is always already infected? A few short sentences, several turns of a phrase, and we are already in a quagmire of deadly incomprehensibility. It will be informative to address these semantic contortions and confusions one at a time.

'Heterosexual sex' is safer sex. In the fusing of gay identity and HIV/AIDS, clearly emblematized in 'GRID' and 'gay plague,' which infects AIDS discourse as a whole, the 'general public' is *a priori* safe. Slippage in meaning occurs here in that behaviors are imbued with identity–as in 'gay sex'/'hetero sex.' How does one read 'gay/hetero sex'? Does 'gay sex' signify all sexual acts between men?/sex between only gay-identified men?/particular behaviors such as anal sex? The feverish denial that anal sex has any place in sex between men and women is exemplary of this slippage. Anal sex is dirty: 'gay sex.' A variety of incoherences and displacements occur when sexual behaviors acquire identity–when they are subsumed, even unconsciously, in an identity matrix. Male-female penetrative vaginal sex, rather than being viewed as a risk behavior *per se,* can be seen as 'heterosexual sex': safer sex. 'Heterosexual sex' is valorized as natural, pure. The various dynamics in this first contortion, a result of slippage and instability in the identity/behavior dichotomy, lead to immense difficulties for prevention. Why use a condom if one is always already safe?

Sex between gay men is necessarily risky. There are several conflicting eddies of meaning here. In the greater power ceded to identity (as opposed to behavior), sex between men who do not identify as gay remains safe–not gay. The obverse is that seropositives are universally presumed to be "infected" with homosexuality. The Centers for Disease Control (CDC) reclassified the epidemiological categories for HIV/AIDS surveillance in the late 1980s largely as a result of the deadly obfuscation that remained pursuant to the risk group story–from "gay men" to "men who have sex with men." Reclassification, of course, is not coextensive with realigning meaning. This epidemiological category shifting provides evidence of the power of the universalizing/minoritizing tension, and also highlights the power and material consequence of how AIDS is represented. The CDC attempted to represent HIV/AIDS anew, to exercise its discursive authority in a dynamic and unstable field of meaning.

Men who have sex with men. Material consequences of the identity-based risk group story are evident in continuing new seroconversions among men who do not identify as gay, but who have sex with other men. For these men who have sex with men, sexual behavior may more likely be anonymous, furtive, guilt-ridden, and practiced under the influence of drugs or alcohol as compared to gay-identified men–though the former certainly have no exclusive dominion along these lines given the ambient homophobic environment in which we all live. Another difficulty for men who do not identify as gay exists in barriers to seeking out, or feeling able to seek out, HIV/AIDS prevention information due to the fear of being "outed" or identified as gay. One risks a puncture in the discursive condom–offered by self-identifying as heterosexual–in seeking out AIDS information and a condom.

'Coming-out positive' is another tragic permutation of the gay-men-are-*a priori*-infected discourse. This construction is founded on the conflation of gay identity and AIDS acting in concert with a master discourse of sexual orientation difference in which gay identity is stigmatized. For gay and proto-gay youth (young people who may not yet identify as gay but who may be located at different points along the developmental trajectory of coming-out)–particularly understood from a minoritizing perspective–seroconversion may, tragically, have become a normative developmental milestone (tombstone?) in the path of gay identity development.

The 'coming-out positive' phenomenon can be seen through a variety of confusions and instabilities. In addition to the conflation of gay identity and AIDS, and the reification of a stigmatized identity, there exists the powerful politics of HIV-positive/HIV-negative–a new discourse of haves and have-nots operationalized by 'the test.' In many ways, for a gay man to be HIV-negative today is to be doubly other–dually stigmatized as both not heterosexual, and as not part of the gay community. This is an untenable position. There also exist immense pressures of survivor guilt, as well as the fear that there will be nothing left of gay culture and community as one knows it (Odets, 1995). Many middle-aged and older gay men have lost their partners, and dozens, even hundreds of friends–their entire social network. This landscape is what a gay or proto-gay youth may envision as his future.

Even as the resources marshaled, often by the gay community itself, only scratch the surface of the need for services for persons living with HIV/AIDS, resources allotted to queer youth in general are even fewer to non-existent. It is comparatively much easier as a gay youth in most locales to procure gay-affirmative support, medical, and psychosocial services by virtue of being seropositive (even as in many places such services are criminally non-existent), than as

HIV-negative. In addition to gaining one access to a community of support, and needed social services, seropositivity may also be romanticized, as in Greg Araki's (1991) *The Living End*–a sort of queer *On the Road* in the age of AIDS. A life of wild abandon, a foreclosed future, may map well onto a present-focused adolescent psyche, sometimes permeated by fantasies of invulnerability.

Be safe. Get tested. Knowledge is power. 'Coming-out positive' is also strongly facilitated by the language of messages espousing testing. I have experienced, anecdotally, in my past clinical practice, several young gay men speak of "the gay, I mean, HIV test" (a perfect conflation of HIV and gay identity). The exhortation for repeated testing can easily be read from the perspective that one takes a test over and over so as eventually to pass (Odets, 1994). An identity/behavior dichotomy–and one in which identity is clearly hegemonic–is strongly operative in that even as HIV may be a function of (unprotected) sexual acts, a stigmatized identity remains deterministic. Why use a condom if seroconversion is an inevitability? Tragically, condoms may become constructed as not-gay, sero-negativity as anti-community. The physical barrier of a condom becomes a discursive barrier to the social support so critical to any youngster–a barrier to community. The 'coming-out positive' phenomenon is exemplary of how differential understandings and conceptualizations of HIV/AIDS may render HIV prevention messages as HIV promotion.

Negatives being positive. The nomenclature of this San Francisco-based support group–along with a host of other playful yet pernicious permutations on the positive/negative theme–represents a new discursive field instantiated by 'the test.' Even as it may acknowledge the needs of HIV-negative gay men and youth for support and community, 'negatives being positive' can easily be read as displacing optimism onto seropositivity. A 'negative' can become positive, then, either through seroconversion or mental conversion. In either case (sero)positivity is aligned as the goal. While 'coming-out positive' may resonate most strongly for gay and proto-gay youth, the problematic dialectics of HIV-positive/HIV-negative operate powerfully across the gay male community as a whole. Even as seropositivity may result in one's being stigmatized, and particularly in areas with smaller and less visible gay populations or lower seroprevalence rates, so may seronegativity result in being ostracized, the familiar feeling of being an outsider—perhaps more likely in larger, urban areas with higher seroprevalence rates and more HIV-related support services.

Vive haya hasta una cura. Be here for the cure. While the message in the bus stops and train stations of San Francisco was largely intended, perhaps, to be read by persons who are HIV-positive, and those already symptomatic, the message itself is symptomatic of overlooking the perspective of an HIV-negative gay man. It is critical that we address the latter—that we develop clarity about who is being targeted by different prevention messages, and as to how these messages may be differentially read—if we are to help HIV-negative gay men and youth stay uninfected. In this message there is espoused a sort of universalistic assumption that we are all HIV-positive—or that it is not proper to affirm the difference in perspective of an HIV-negative gay man. As if our HIV-negative gay and proto-gay (and proto-HIV-positive?) youth needed further mystification, and further impetus to become HIV-positive, with "the cure" on the horizon, the deluge of HIV becomes a spring rain. Celebrate. Feel it. Get wet. Why wear a raincoat?

Men—Use a condom or beat it. Use a condom every time. Another consequence of the already infected gay body is the omission of the possibility that two HIV-negative men might reasonably choose to fuck without a condom: They must proceed as if HIV-positive. This results in part from operating as if we were in the pre-HIV-test epidemic when there was no way to discern seropositivity. It also results from internalization of a heteronormative minoritizing perspective which equates gay identity with seropositivity. The consequence is that we are nullifying a major motivation for using a condom in the first place: one may sustain condom use in general so as to be able to enjoy what is now termed unprotected sex with a partner known to be HIV-negative (Odets, 1994).

Know your partner. This much-invoked message implies that within the confines of a relationship, even more a presumably monogamous relationship, "knowing" is tantamount to safer sex. It has been empirically demonstrated that a great deal of serotransmission occurs in couples, as condom use is more inconsistent than in sex practiced outside of a relationship (see Hospers & Kok, 1995).

Tragically, repeated unprotected sex with the known partner who may already be HIV-positive may be a reliable and efficient means of serotransmission. When one transposes the meaning of 'know your partner,' and of monogamy, into a 17-year-old's world view, where a week may be going steady, and a month a long-term relationship, the violence wrought by this message is further revealed. 'Know your partner' is imbued with existing messages which emphasize identity over behavior, and offer identity as a basis of prevention. It is also laden with moralistic contortions which construct 'promiscuous sex'—as opposed to unprotected sex—as responsible for HIV transmission. Here slippage in the discursive condom—subscribing to the fallacy of relying on identity as either not-gay or not-promiscuous as a safer sex technique—can again be seen to enable HIV transmission.

'Safer' partners have risky sex. Another manifestation of slippage in meaning occurs among gay men along the HIV-positive/HIV-negative divide. This is exemplified in more than one published confessional (Warner, 1995b), where a knowledgeable and otherwise 'safer' sexual actor reports an incident of unprotected anal sex. One aspect of such a sexual slip is a discursive slip that occurs because safer sex is always imbricated with disease. For a gay man to use (or demand that a partner use) a condom, is to invoke contagion: If one needs to have safer sex, one must be infected. Similarly, if one's partner does not invoke the need for a condom, he must be 'safe'—HIV-negative—in a teleological and self-confirmatory argument.

If one is HIV-positive, one may then assume one's partner, who also does not mention condoms, is also seropositive. Communication around sex, already so difficult, is made vastly more distorted and loaded in the unstable and contestational field of the language of AIDS—particularly as manifested in the HIV-positive/HIV-negative dichotomy. What results from this instability is a clear double bind: In calling for safer sex (behavior), one becomes marked (and identified) as 'risky.'

While the problems of prevention reside in part in the strong undertow of identity—its discursive hegemony over behavior—shifting to a universalizing perspective is not the solution. The even minor effort of the federal government to address HIV by marketing prevention *en masse*—sending a flyer to every American household, marketing public service announcements to mass audiences—can be seen to operate from a universalizing standpoint. Such universalization, however, becomes synonymous with heteronormativity. Proto-gay and gay youth are written out of prevention. This is further supported by a federal ban on funding for any education that might be seen as "promoting" or "condoning" homosexuality, in a Helmsian (per)version of free speech.

Mass public health campaigns defy the existence of different populations, with different comprehensions and discourses surrounding HIV/AIDS—they ignore the existence of differing understandings of AIDS, and of different subject positions. Recent research, however, has underscored the need to differentially target youth and adults; gay, lesbian, bisexual, and heterosexual youth; African American, Latino/a, Asian American, and white youth (Aggleton, O'Reilly, Slutkin, & Davies, 1994; Icard, 1992; Jemmott, Jemmott, & Fong, 1992). The discourse of Black gay men, for example, several researchers have found, around sex, AIDS, identity, and disease, may be quite different from that of white gay men, with differential ramifications for prevention (Icard, 1992; Mays, Cochran, Belliga, & Smith, 1992).

A related problem of a universalistic prevention discourse is that in focusing too narrowly on body parts and sexual dynamics, glorious though they may be, one may omit the powerful ground of stigma, of racism, homophobia, sexism, heterosexism, ageism, poverty, and other forms of marginalization that are strongly implicated in the epidemiology of HIV. More difficult than adopting either a minoritizing or a universalizing position is cultivation of the ability to read prevention discourse from both perspectives. This enables us to see how HIV prevention messages may be unintelligible and, worse, counterproductive.

In addition to incoherences in HIV prevention discourse, one can glean competing conceptualizations of sexuality, and of AIDS, in the arguments of those who would disallow AIDS education for young people—indeed who would block federal funding for HIV prevention overall. There exist federal statutes barring funding for any messages that "promote" or "condone" homosexuality. The radical right seems to operate with an identity-based concept of heterosexuality as sealed off from gay/lesbian–a minoritizing position. At the same time, universalism is evident in a constant obsession with contagion. Merely mentioning the word gay is tantamount to infecting (read: heterosexual) youth. Invoking AIDS is likewise the first step to 'promiscuity' and infection. With the instability of meaning underscoring these positions, HIV prevention is fraught with the potential for differential projects for control over representation and meaning, and in the service of different ends. What has been characterized as a war of prevention–alternatively practiced as a war on prevention–must be fought on the level of meaning and representation (how we present and communicate about AIDS), as well as on the biomedical level–as if the two could be so neatly subdivided. Strategic intervention on the level of discourse and representation is a substantive and essential survival strategy for HIV-negative gay men in the 1990s.

NEW PREVENTION STRATEGIES FOR THE 1990s

While we cannot permanently inoculate ourselves against either homophobia or heteronormativity–there is no vaccine–we can seek out and anticipate the incoherences and the obfuscations in our prevention and education messages, as well as in the arguments of our detractors. We can engage directly in the contentious field of representation. Representation, writes Hall (1982, 64), "implies the active work of selecting and presenting, of structuring and shaping: not merely the transmitting of already-existing meaning, but the more active labor of *making things mean*" [emphasis added]. My focus has been that of unpacking what are in effect discursive condoms–apocryphal prophylaxes for HIV–enabled by competing representations of AIDS. A discursive condom is a fallacious and frequently ineffective prevention strategy based solely on linguistic, semantic, or identity-based constructions.

Understanding the motivations that may support different representations of HIV/AIDS, and discerning the ways in which our prevention messages may be infected with counterproductive meanings, are integral to a strategy of engaging in the confrontational sphere of meaning-making. As in many other arenas, "In the representations of AIDS the messages most likely to reach their destination are messages already there" (Bersani, 1988, 210). Nevertheless, we need not buy into and recycle heteronormative assumptions, nor must we adhere blindly to unilaterally minoritizing or universalizing points of view.

Another integral aspect of a prevention strategy that acknowledges the power of language and meaning, and meaning-making, is a critical awareness of oneself, including one's own understanding of sexuality and HIV/AIDS. To engage in the domain of language and meaning-making we must challenge and dialogue about our own identities and conceptualizations of what it is to be gay, lesbian, bisexual, queer, transgender, or heterosexual, what it means to be HIV-positive or HIV-negative, and what it means to be 'safe' and 'unsafe,' in the 1990s.

We must acknowledge the minefield constituted by HIV and fostered by historical tensions in discourse regarding sexuality, identity, and disease. In approaching HIV/AIDS as a discursive phenomenon, however—in risking a puncture in the discursive condom—I hazard being labeled and ostracized as uncaring. I am risking accusations of counterproductively breeding more confusion and indeterminacy through a form of mental masturbation. In the not so new, individualistic language of reasoned action somewhat misleadingly layered onto HIV prevention—*Staying Negative.—It's Not Automatic. Think About It. Talk About It.*—I have determined this to be an acceptable level of risk.

REFERENCES

Aggleton, P., O'Reilly, K., Slutkin, G. & Davies, P. (1994). Risking everything? Risk behavior, behavior change, and AIDS. *Science, 265,* 341-345.

Araki, G. (Director/Producer). (1991). *The living end* [Film]. (Available on video, Strand release/Despearate pictures, Academy entertainment, catalog # 1710).

Bersani, L. (1988). Is the rectum a grave? In D. Crimp (Ed.), *AIDS: Cultural analysis/cultural activism.* Massachusetts: MIT Press.

Fleming, P. (1996). *Youth and AIDS: A White House report.* Washington, DC: U.S. Government Printing Office.

Foucault, M. (1978). *The history of sexuality: An introduction.* New York: Vintage Books.

Gilman, S. (1988). AIDS and syphilis: The iconography of disease. In D. Crimp (Ed.), *AIDS: Cultural analysis/cultural activism.* Massachusetts: MIT Press.

Goffman, E. (1963). *Stigma: Notes on the management of a spoiled identity.* New York: Jason Aronson.

Hall, S. (1982). The rediscovery of 'ideology': Return of the repressed in media studies. In M. Gurevitch (Ed.), *Culture, society and the media*. London: Methuen Press.

Hart, G., & Boulton, M. (1995). Sexual behavior in gay men: Towards a sociology of risk. In P. Aggleton, P. Davies & G. Hart (Eds.), *AIDS: Safety, sexuality and risk*. London: Taylor and Francis.

Hospers, H., & Kok, G. (1995). Determinants of safe and risk-taking sexual behavior among gay men: A review. *AIDS Education and Prevention, 7*(1), 74-97.

Icard, L. (1992). Preventing AIDS among black gay men and black gay and heterosexual male intravenous drug users. *Social Work, 37*(5), 440-445.

Jemmott, J., Jemmott, L., & Fong, G. (1992). Reductions in HIV risk-associated sexual behaviors among black male adolescents. *American Journal of Public Health, 82*(3), 372-377.

Johnston, W. I. (1995). *HIV-negative: How the uninfected are affected by AIDS*. New York: Plenum Press.

Mays, V., Cochran, S., Belliga, G., & Smith, R. (1992). The language of black gay men's sexual behavior: Implications for AIDS risk reduction. *Journal of Sex Research, 29*(3), 425-434.

Neisen, J. H. (1990). Heterosexism: Redefining homophobia in the 1990s. *Journal of Gay & Lesbian Psychotherapy, 1*(3), 21-35.

Nelkin, D. & Gilman, S. (1988). Placing blame for devastating disease. *Social Research, 55*(3), 361-378.

Odets, W. (1994). AIDS education and harm reduction: Psychological approaches for the 21st century. *AIDS and Public Policy Journal, 9*(1), 3-15.

Odets, W. (1995). *In the shadow of the epidemic: Being HIV-negative in the age of AIDS*. Durham, North Carolina: Duke University Press.

Rofes, E. (1996). *Reviving the tribe: Regenerating gay men's sexuality and culture in the ongoing epidemic*. New York: The Harrington Park Press.

Sadownick, D. (1995). Beyond condoms. *LA Weekly*, (June 16-22), 22-29.

Sedgwick, E. K. (1990). *Epistemology of the closet*. Berkeley: University of California Press.

Shernoff, M. (1996, February). [Personal Communication]. New York.

Stall, R., Ekstrand, M., Pollack, L., McKusick, L., & Coates, T. J. (1990). Relapse from safer sex: The next challenge for AIDS prevention efforts. *Journal of Acquired Immune Deficiency Syndromes, 3*, 1181-7.

Warner, M. (1995a). Negative attitude. *Voice Literary Supplement*, (September), 25-27.

Warner, M. (1995b). Unsafe: Why gay men are having risky sex. *The Village Voice*, January 31, 33-36.

Weinberg, G. (1973). *Society and the healthy homosexual*. New York: Anchor.

New Drugs and HIV Risk Taking: Observations of Therapists Who Work with HIV-Negative Gay Men

Arthur Fox

SUMMARY. Many workers in HIV-prevention and mental health have feared that publicity surrounding new drugs for treating HIV would cause HIV-negative gay men to lapse from safer sex. However, a recent informal survey of health workers and therapists in New York City suggests that although information about the new drugs has shifted the thinking of many negative men, it hasn't changed their behavior a great deal as yet. Anecdotal evidence of minor behavior change is described, along with medical data concerning how dangerous unsafe sex with an infected person undergoing combination drug therapy may be. *[Article copies available for a fee from The Haworth Document Delivery Service: 1-800-342-9678. E-mail address: getinfo@haworth.com]*

Splashy media coverage of new medical treatments for HIV and AIDS over the past year has made many therapists, researchers, and prevention workers brace themselves for a new wave of "unsafe

---

Arthur Fox is a doctoral candidate in clinical psychology at City College of New York.

Address correspondence to: Arthur Fox, Clinical Psychology NAC 8/101, City College of New York, 138th Street and Convent Avenue, New York, NY 10027.

[Haworth co-indexing entry note]: "New Drugs and HIV Risk Taking: Observations of Therapists Who Work with HIV-Negative Gay Men." Fox, Arthur. Co-published simultaneously in *Journal of Gay & Lesbian Social Services* (The Haworth Press, Inc.) Vol. 8, No. 1, 1998, pp. 103-108; and: *The HIV-Negative Gay Man: Developing Strategies for Survival and Emotional Well-Being* (ed: Steven Ball) The Haworth Press, Inc., 1998, pp. 103-108; and: *The HIV-Negative Gay Man: Developing Strategies for Survival and Emotional Well-Being* (ed: Steven Ball) The Harrington Park Press, an imprint of The Haworth Press, Inc., 1998, pp. 103-108. Single or multiple copies of this article are available for a fee from The Haworth Document Delivery Service [1-800-342-9678, 9:00 a.m. - 5:00 p.m. (EST). E-mail address: getinfo@haworth.com].

103

sex" among HIV-negative gay men. Because new combination therapies often drastically reduce the serum concentration of the HIV virus in many people—often seeming to eliminate the virus's presence in the bloodstream entirely—concerns have recently been expressed that gay men, both infected and uninfected, are likely to revert to their old ways (e.g., Rotello, 1997). Positive men may believe they are no longer likely to transmit the virus to their partners through sex. Negative men may believe that becoming infected with HIV is now an insignificant—and even reversible—health threat.

This paper reviews the fictions and realities underlying the expectations of both sexually active gay men and the professionals trying to help them survive. It looks at the behavior changes that mental health workers "on the front line" have actually observed in HIV-negative gay men over the past year. It also discusses the medical evidence concerning the health threats that these behavior changes represent.

An informal canvassing of a nonrandom sample of HIV prevention workers in New York City in January 1997 suggests that technologies like the protease inhibitor drugs haven't, as yet, precipitated widespread changes in sexual behavior. These prevention workers who were asked what, if any, changes in thinking and behavior around safer sex they had observed over the past year in the populations they work closely with, concurred that whatever increase in unsafe sex has occured over the past year appears to be largely among men who were already practicing safer sex inconsistently. The new drugs, and the idea that they may mean that HIV infection is a chronic and treatable condition rather than a fatal one, is for many HIV-negative gay men another ambiguous clue in the system of wishes and compromises that shape their safer-sex decisions.

Men who strongly want to have anal sex without condoms may find themselves using the optimistic reports about the efficacy of protease inhibitors as part of their repertoire of rationalizations. "For the ones who want to deny, the protease drugs just give them another excuse," said Joyce Hunter, DSW, of the HIV Center for Clinical and Behavioral Studies in New York City.

Donald Jackson, HIV coordinator for New York's Gay Men of African Descent, a social and educational organization, agrees that if there is an increase in unsafe sex over the past year, it's among those men who were having difficulty staying safe even before the new drugs came along. Jackson says that among the men he counsels, factors like feeling caught up in the moment, or feeling that infection is inevitable, influence decisions around unsafe sex more powerfully than any incipient belief that AIDS has become a manageable disease. This may be, he says, because African-American men may be less likely to believe that they will have access to expensive and protracted medical treatments should they become infected.

Moreover, Jackson says, Black gay men as a group may be suspicious of drugs, and of the "medical establishment" in general (Jones, 1981), and may be less likely than white men to believe that doctors and medications can help them if they are, or become, infected. Therefore HIV-positive Black men, Jackson says, may be less likely to have been tested, and to know that they are HIV-positive, than white men. This, Jackson says, can lead to a kind of denial, that may result in a failure to communicate with partners about possible risk. A common strategy among those who suspect that they are infected, Jackson says, is "Until I get sick and have to go to the hospital I'm going to get my groove on, I'm going to get mine."

If the new drugs haven't changed actual behavior a great deal among the clients of the professionals interviewed for this paper, they have, nevertheless, changed the way many HIV-negative gay men think about sex, risk, and their future.

William Johnston, a therapist in Boston and author of the book *HIV-Negative: How the Uninfected Are Affected by AIDS* (1995), believes that the news about AIDS treatment will be a less powerful influence on sexual behavior than the subtle psychological issues that already are undermining gay men's efforts to stay safe. Johnston believes that one of the most powerful of these forces is negative gay men's unconscious desire to feel and express solidarity with positive gay men—to not exclude, and to feel more a part of the fold of gay life. Does the belief that new drugs make HIV a chronic illness in itself help to close this gap? If it does, Johnston says, it doesn't seem to have entered into the sexual decisions of the men in his HIV-negative groups.

John Grimaldi, a psychiatrist who directs the AIDS Center at St.Vincent's Hospital in New York, says that if the new drugs are having an effect on the safer-sex thinking of HIV-negative men, it may, paradoxically, be increasing safety behavior. The fact that the idea of becoming infected feels less catastrophic now than it felt a year ago, Grimaldi says, is making some negative men "more able to do what it takes to protect themselves. The possibility that failing and becoming infected now won't be a death sentence is enabling them to muster the enthusiasm for helping themselves."

Therapist Michael Shernoff says he is seeing the effects of the new treatments on both the thinking and the sexual behavior of the HIV-negative men in his practice in New York City. For many, the change is a response to the fact that protease inhibitors may be prolonging the lives of positive men. Many negative men who formerly wouldn't date positive men out of fear of loss, Shernoff says, now believe they may have "ten or fifteen good years" with a positive partner. The negative men in his practice who still won't go out with men who are positive, Shernoff says, tend to be those who have already buried lovers.

Shernoff's clients–those who are positive and on the new drugs, and those who are in love with men who are–have fairly good reason to be optimistic about the future at this point. Although the drugs are fairly new, radical improvements in viral load and health seem to be holding up fairly well. Although the drugs work better for some patients than for others–and although in some patients they don't appear to work well at all–many people who have been on the treatments show sustained improvement.

But because very few patients have been on these treatments for more than two years, the drugs' ability to minimize the action of the virus over the long term is unknown. Researchers say that even when an infected person's blood HIV levels have been reduced to undetectable levels, the virus may still be "hiding out" in areas of the body that the drugs are unable to reach–areas like the cerebro-spinal fluid and the lymph tissue (Boswell, 1997). Because HIV may reside in these areas for many years, researchers can't begin to speculate that the virus has been "eliminated" from an infected person's body until blood levels have been below detection range for at least four or five years.

Everyone seems to know someone who knows someone who has recently decided to have unprotected anal sex with an HIV-positive man whose "viral load" has been reduced to undetectable levels by protease inhibitors. There appears to be, among some gay men, an intuitive assumption that when sensitive chemical tests can no longer detect the presence of HIV in the blood, this means there is little or no chance of passing the virus to a sexual partner through semen.

This is incorrect. Researchers say that active virus may well be present in the semen of people whose blood appears to be virus-free (Boswell, 1997). Nevertheless, the idea that unprotected penetration with a positive partner now entails "less risk" appears to be widespread. In Shernoff's practice, this kind of thinking is cropping up most in negative men with positive partners. A partner's reduced viral load, coupled with a belief that the partner "has no precum," can tip the scales such that these men are willing to be penetrated by their partners without ejaculation. These men are "fairly sophisticated consumers," Shernoff says, and express some anxiety that this could be risky. But unprotected penetration gives these men a feeling of closeness with their partner that justifies the gamble.

Other changes that Shernoff has seen among negative men is an increased willingness to have oral sex to ejaculation; for many, the belief that a partner, if infected, may be less infectious—coupled with the not-entirely-conscious belief that there may be a "morning after" pill to take in the event that infection occurs—makes whatever rules they have against taking semen in the mouth seem less urgent.

Medically, both these wishful beliefs are unfounded. Researchers studying HIV's response to protease inhibitors say that there is no evidence that the new drugs reduce the danger in viral transmission (Boswell, 1997). Because the structure of the virus changes in response to the new medications, it is possible that a person on combination therapy can infect a sexual partner with a form of the virus that is more lethal—more resistant to medication—than the one he himself is infected with.

As for the "morning after pill," although studies trying to create documentable "seroreversion" in newly infected persons are currently in the works, there is no evidence yet that exposure to HIV can be undone at any point post-hoc (Boswell, 1997). Although researchers and clinicians are seeing different effects from the introduction of new treatment technologies over the past year, they agree that negative men's decisions around sexual risk are based less on objective information than on desire.

Thus, while it is essential that HIV-negative gay men have accurate data on the implications of the new HIV drugs for infectivity and survival, it may be more urgent at this point for negative men to get help understanding the feelings that motivate them, consciously or unconsciously, to put themselves at risk for infection. Factors like survivor guilt and the identity needs attendant to sex are harder to talk about than thoughts about how well AIDS drugs work, but when these issues are articulated by therapists, feelings around these issues become more manageable. "Sometimes just naming it is enough to alert people," Johnston says.

REFERENCES

Boswell, S. (1997). "HIV/AIDS update." Address to the Opening Plenary Session of the National Lesbian and Gay Health Association Annual Conference. Atlanta, GA.

Johnston, W. (1995). *HIV negative: How the uninfected are affected by AIDS.* New York: Insight Books.

Jones, J. (1981). Bad blood: The Tuskeege syphilis experiment. New York: Free Press.

Rotello, G. (1997). *Sexual ecology: AIDS and the destiny of gay men.* New York: Dutton.

Index

Notes: For the *Journal of Gay & Lesbian Social Services* co-published version
of this book: the page numbers for subjects indexed from the Foreword
are enclosed in square brakets, e.g., *xiii[xvii]*.

Page numbers preceded by *mentioned* denotes intermittent discussion
of subject on each inclusive page.

T - #0251 - 101024 - C0 - 212/152/8 [10] - CB - 9780789005229 - Gloss Lamination